Staying Human during Residency Training: How to Survive and Thrive after Medical School

SIXTH EDITION

The ultimate survival guide for medical students, interns, residents, and fellows, *Staying Human during Residency Training* provides time-tested advice and the latest information on every aspect of a resident's life – from choosing a residency program to coping with stress, enhancing self-care, and protecting personal and professional relationships.

Allan D. Peterkin, MD, provides hundreds of tips on how to cope with sleep deprivation, time pressures, and ethical and legal issues. This sixth edition is not only updated to reflect the latest research and resources, but also features new material on current issues in residency training, including social media use, patient-centered care, the medical humanities, and the "hidden curriculum" of residency. Presenting practical antidotes to cynicism, careerism, and burnout, Peterkin also offers guidance on fostering more empathic connection with patients and deepening relationships with colleagues, friends, and family.

Acknowledged by thousands of doctors across North America as an invaluable resource, *Staying Human during Residency Training* has helped to shape notions of trainee well-being for medical educators worldwide. Offering wise, compassionate, and professional counsel, this new edition again shows why it is required reading for medical students and new physicians pursuing postgraduate training.

ALLAN D. PETERKIN is a practicing psychiatrist and a professor in the Departments of Psychiatry and Community and Family Medicine at the University of Toronto, where he also heads the Health, Arts and Humanities Program.

Praise for Previous Editions

"Through most of this century physicians have looked back on their internship and residency years as a painful but necessary maturation ritual. Once out of residency, they quickly forget or at least deny, how much damage – depression, burn-out, marriage breakdown, alcoholism and suicide – was wrought during the process. Allan Peterkin ... provides a useful guide for self-preservation and well-being. It should be required reading for all graduating medical students."
Bruce P. Squires, MD, PhD, former editor-in-chief,
Canadian Medical Association Journal

"This guide should be required reading for each intern beginning residency and also for each and every residency program director in North America."
Aliye Runyan, Medical Education Team Chair,
American Medical Student Association (AMSA), and Sonia Lazreg,
AMSA/Committee of Interns and Residents Health Justice Fellow

"*Staying Human during Residency Training* is an important reminder: that humane treatment – of oneself and fellow residents, as well as our patients – is what makes a good doctor, and that one cannot have empathy without good self-caretaking. That is a lesson we can all afford to review."
Sonya Rasminsky, MD, *CIR News*

"An excellent resource for residents at any stage in their training."
The Canadian Association of Internes and Residents

"There is no area in a resident's life that Dr. Peterkin doesn't tackle: finances, substance abuse, fellowship options, foreign, gay, and disabled students, ethical and legal considerations, study tips and support groups. It's the ultimate how-to book for all apprentice doctors and its commonsense approach makes it a mandatory trouble-shooter."
Elaine McNinch, *Family Practice*

"This catalog of indispensable advice can help residents at all stages of training. Read it today, and pass it on!"
Wayne M. Sotile, PhD, author of *Letting Go of What's Holding You Back!* and *The Resilient Physician*

"Dr Peterkin is Canada's expert on residency health and sustainability. Thorough, practical, and contemporary, *Staying Human during Residency* is a must-read for all resident physicians."
Dr Derek Puddester, associate professor of psychiatry,
and director of the Faculty of Wellness Program, University of Ottawa

"Chock-full of all kinds of information that is pertinent, if not essential, to residents, including innumerable survival tips and suggestions. Dr Peterkin offers a penetrating and far-ranging, yet humane, perspective and has not lost sight of the 'person within,' in contrast to attitudes common in academic medical centres of today. This book will go a long way toward alleviating much of the worry and demoralization among contemporary residents, as well as their partners or spouses. A copy should be stuffed into the pocket of every resident physician."
Michael Myers, MD, author of *Doctors' Marriages: A Look at Problems and Their Solutions* and co-author, *The Handbook of Physician Health*

Staying Human during Residency Training

How to Survive and Thrive after Medical School

SIXTH EDITION

Allan D. Peterkin

UNIVERSITY OF TORONTO PRESS
Toronto Buffalo London

Library and Archives Canada Cataloguing in Publication

Peterkin, Allan D., author
Staying human during residency training : how to survive and thrive after
medical school / Allan D. Peterkin. – Sixth edition.

Includes bibliographical references and index.
ISBN 978-1-4426-2914-1 (paper)

1. Residents (Medicine) – Canada – Life skills guides. 2. Residents
(Medicine) – United States – Life skills guides. I. Title.

R840.P48 2016   610.71'55   C2016-900391-4

University of Toronto Press acknowledges the financial assistance to its
publishing program of the Canada Council for the Arts and the Ontario Arts
Council, an agency of the Government of Ontario.

**Canada Council
for the Arts**

**Conseil des Arts
du Canada**

ONTARIO ARTS COUNCIL
CONSEIL DES ARTS DE L'ONTARIO

an Ontario government agency
un organisme du gouvernement de l'Ontario

Funded by the
Government
of Canada

Financé par le
gouvernement
du Canada

In memory of my father, Dr David Peterkin,
A true renaissance man.

For Dr Edith K. Peterkin,
My aunt, mentor, and friend.

Nothing will sustain you more potently than the power to recognize in your humdrum routine, as perhaps it may be thought, the true poetry of life – the poetry of the commonplace, of the ordinary man, of the plain, toil-worn woman, with their loves and their joys, their sorrows and their griefs. The comedy, too, of life will be spread before you, and nobody laughs more often than the doctor at the pranks Puck plays upon the Titanias and the Bottoms among his patients. The humorous side is really almost as frequently turned towards him as the tragic. Lift up one hand to heaven and thank your stars if they have given you the proper sense to enable you to appreciate the inconceivably droll situations in which we catch our fellow creatures. Unhappily, this is one of the free gifts of the gods, unevenly distributed, not bestowed on all, or on all in equal proportions. In undue measure it is not without risk, and in any case in the doctor it is better appreciated by the eye than expressed on the tongue. Hilarity and good humour, a breezy cheerfulness, a nature "sloping toward the sunny side," as Lowell has it, help enormously both in the study and in the practice of medicine. To many of a sombre and sour disposition it is hard to maintain good spirits amid the trials and tribulations of the day, and yet it is an unpardonable mistake to go about among patients with a long face.

– Sir William Osler, The student life.
In *Aequanimitas with Other Addresses*, 3rd ed., Blakiston, New York, 1953: 397–423

Contents

Foreword

Residency may be the most difficult years of a physician's life: unknown information seems to overwhelm even the most studious; there is a never-ending battle with sleep deprivation; we juggle work, exams, and research as we transition into new roles with our families and friends and the rest of our lives. Added to these expected challenges are others that may tempt us to become disillusioned and discouraged: endless demands, insufficient time, difficult personalities, tedious rounds, and decisions that do not always seem to be in the best interests of our patients. Even more disheartening are the ever-present reports of poor coping mechanisms used by trainees and even physician suicide. Given this reality, the sixth edition of *Staying Human during Residency Training* is a refreshingly honest and unique guide designed to provide resources for optimism, humanism, and resilience.

At the American Medical Student Association (AMSA), we pride ourselves on being a resource for the overall wellness of physicians-in-training. From our institutes on Narrative Medicine and Medical Humanities, and our fourth-year rotation on reflective transformation (HEART) to prior collaborations with the Committee of Interns and Residents (CIR) to reduce medical work hours in the interests of both trainees and our patients, we provide tools and advocate for an improved system.

The Canadian Federation of Medical Students (CFMS) similarly prioritizes our efforts to ensure student wellness through direct engagement with our members and with national organizations that share similar goals. The CFMS Wellness Committee has rapidly grown in membership and scope over the past few years; our work with our partners aims to first better understand wellness needs and to provide corresponding services and restructured learning environments where necessary.

Staying Human during Residency Training fits with our shared organizational values and is an excellent addition to the toolbox of resources available to help trainees not simply to survive the path to becoming a doctor but to thrive along the way. The sixth edition of the book provides insight into areas of critical importance: basic mental health skills for all physicians, patient safety and quality improvement, the physician as patient, cultivating resilience, and resources for patient advocacy, especially for marginalized populations. This edition also includes topics such as reflective capacity, making the hidden curriculum explicit, effectively navigating hierarchies, and practicing inter-professionalism.

This guide should be required reading for each intern beginning residency, and also for each and every residency program director in North America – to be more aware of their residents' burdens and needs. We envision a healthcare system where all trainees engage fully in their education and patient care while preserving their own humanity.

We are excited to see this invaluable classic become even more widely circulated among US and Canadian programs to encourage residency directors and residents alike to implement a more humanistic perspective within their training programs.

Staying Human during Residency Training will be helpful in achieving this reality, as it bolsters individual resilience while advocating for medical education to improve and nurture its trainees.

Aliye Runyan, MD
Graduate Trustee, AMSA
Resident, Dept. of Obstetrics
Wayne State University /
   Detroit Medical Center
Detroit, MI, USA

Jesse Kancir, MSc, MD
Immediate Past-President, Canadian
   Federation of Medical Students
   and Gynecology
2014–2015 Chevening Scholar;
   MPhil Public Policy Candidate
University of Cambridge
Cambridge, UK

Introduction

One of the smartest things a medical student, resident, fellow, or faculty member could do in their entire career is read and reflect on the wisdom in this very practical book. The Faculty Wellness Program at our school works with several hundred medical students and physicians every year and routinely recommends *Staying Human during Residency Training* in our courses, workshops, lectures, and coaching sessions. Simply put, you will increase and enhance your resiliency and sustainability by investing some time in Dr Peterkin's thoughtful and relevant book.

Residency training is a delightful time in many ways. Residents enjoy a tremendous growth in their knowledge and skills, their competence and confidence as clinicians rapidly develops, their teaching and learning skills mature, and their appreciation of and ability to influence the complex healthcare system begins to reach a stage of mastery. All of this allows them to do what patients and communities need them to do: promote health, minimize the effects of illness, disease, and disability, and make their communities better places to enjoy life and family. That said, residency can also pose a health hazard.

Patients are presenting with more complex needs and more acute care issues; healthcare teams struggle to find time to work on team identity, development, and conflict management; expectations regarding professionalism and comportment are shifting, with little time dedicated to skill and attitude development; and the sheer academic demands for all healthcare providers continue to rise. Mix in normal adult development (sexuality, identity, self-growth), possible marriages / divorces, parenting / caring for ageing parents, financial pressures, and a normal need for free time, recreation, and play ... well, this is a phase of life that has its own crucial demands.

So let's be very practical ... We need help to stay human during this challenging time of our professional development. Perhaps the best advice is to take advantage of as many tools, resources, mentors, coaches, colleagues, friends, and family members as possible. This new edition is very practical and will highlight those resources and strategies that can bring immediate benefit to your life. It also contains poems and narratives actually written by trainees and new information on areas often neglected in residency programs: the challenges of new media, patient safety, the hidden curriculum, the role of the medical humanities in developing reflective capacity and in exploring social justice, and a delineation of mental health competencies ALL doctors should possess if they want to provide humanistic care.

For students, there are excellent tips on preparing for residency. This is one of the biggest transitions you will face in your professional career! Read up on how to choose a humane residency, how to recognize the strengths and challenges of a residency program, and how to take control of the transition of residency in a manner that will keep you healthy and well for many years.

For residents, bear in mind that the vast majority of physicians are healthy and resilient, and for good reason: they brought strengths and talents with them into medicine that promoted their academic and personal success. Hopefully, this new edition of *Staying Human* will increase the dialogue on wellness among colleagues on both sides of the border.

Nurture and sustain your strengths carefully! Dr Peterkin will coach you on how to monitor your physical and mental health, and how to juggle your multiple demands and bosses, and will even help you prepare for the transition to independent practice. His advice is immediately applicable and practical. I would urge you to use your experience along with the advice in this book to also nurture and support your colleagues (and even your supervisors)!

Finally, for faculty members, hold tight to your memories of life as a resident and the normal (and excessive) challenges you faced and managed. Bear in mind that the healthcare system has changed and evolved since we were in training and we may not fully appreciate the new tensions and challenges our trainees face. While we need to help our trainees achieve competence and strive for excellence, we also need to model a professional life that is sustainable, meaningful, and mindful of the joy of caring.

Our humanity is what brought us to medicine. Our human experiences with our patients and colleagues are what sustain us. By being mindful of how to stay human, often by implementing many of Dr Peterkin's practical strategies, we can support each other, enjoy a rich and vibrant practice, and give our patients the empathic and genuine care they deserve.

Derek Puddester, CEC MD MEd FRCP(C)
Dr Puddester is the lead editor of the RCPSC's CanMEDS
   Physician Health Guide and co-author of the RCPSC's
   Time Management Guide. He also produced *Carpe Diem*
   (a physician resiliency documentary), and was the project
   lead for ePhysicianHealth.com and eWorkplaceHealth.com.
See www.puddester.com for more information on his
   publications and coaching seminars.

Acknowledgments

Thank you to my teachers, students, residents, colleagues, and patients who have taught me so much over the years and to my family who make sure my own life stays in balance.

Thanks to the University of Toronto Press for encouraging me to update *Staying Human* (on a regular basis over 20 years!) so that it remains relevant to new generations of future healers.

Thanks to Dr Derek Puddester, one of the world's experts on physician health, for his warm feedback about the book and his Introduction.

Thanks to Dr Aliye Runyan from the American Medical Student Association and Dr Jesse Kancir from the Canadian Federation of Medical Students for their thoughtful Foreword.

Thanks to Dr Ian Williams, one of the founders of the graphic medicine movement worldwide (see www.graphicmedicine.org), who generously put out a call to his colleagues for illustrations of the trainee experience and then submitted some panels himself from his own training days. This led to the inclusion of compelling visual works by Monica Lalanda, Janet Lee-Evoy, Ryan Montoya, Linda Chang Qu, Alex Thomas, and Ian Williams in the e-version of this book.

Thanks to BOA Editions, publishers *of Body Language – Poems of the Medical Training Experience*, who allowed me to reprint wonderful poems on residency from that collection by Richard Berlin, David Kopacz, Mairi Leining, and Emily Transue.

Thank you to residents Paul D'Alessandro, Mehr-Afarin Hosseini, Sara Raiser, Raphael Rush, and Alex Saltman for contributing personal narratives and coping tips directly from their real-time residency experiences across specialties and from all over North America.

Each edition of *Staying Human during Residency Training* has been deeply enriched by hands-on feedback from the talented men and women this book was written for in the first place.

Allan Peterkin
2016
Toronto
www.drpeterkin.com

Staying Human during Residency Training:
How to Survive and Thrive after Medical School

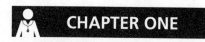

CHAPTER ONE

Body and Soul:
The Risks, Challenges, and Incredible
Opportunities of Residency Training

Congratulations on finishing medical school and welcome to residency!

Post-grad medical training can be stressful, but it also provides many opportunities for great personal and professional development. Interns and residents are not fragile people; you are bright, compassionate, and dedicated men and women who are eager to learn. Although residency presents multiple challenges and stressors, it also affords the opportunity for young doctors to develop resilience and coping skills that will serve them throughout their careers. Along with medical students, residents make up approximately one-fifth of the physician workforce in the United States and Canada. It is striking, however, that some of the character traits that lead many people toward a career in medicine are also predictors of possible struggles and impairment.[1,2,3] High levels of responsibility, intense contact with people, time restrictions, role uncertainty and transition (i.e., from student to neophyte professional), sleep deprivation, and social isolation are linked to stress in any profession. Although residency is a much better place to be than when the first edition of this book came out, significant stressors are still present in postgraduate medical education. In addition, residents must deal directly with suffering, fear, death, uncertainty, and problem patients and staff.[4] In these circumstances, it is not surprising that they suffer varying degrees of stress-related symptoms, however healthy they may be on entering residency. What's different today is that burnout is not seen as an inevitable byproduct of training. Resilience and compassion for self and others are its antidotes, and you'll learn how to cultivate both throughout these chapters.

Table 1.1 Your Responsibilities as a Resident or Intern

---

1 Admit new patients.
2 Visit and examine all patients on your team each morning.
3 Attend working rounds.
4 Present your cases, update chart notes.
5 Teach and supervise medical students.
6 Communicate with other care team members (including nurses, the pharmacist,
   social worker, ward clerk, physician assistant).
7 Order appropriate imaging studies and lab work.
8 Request appropriate consultations.
9 Attend follow-up and sign-out rounds.
10 Plan discharges and dictate discharge notes.
11 Arrange discharge meds and out-patient follow up.
12 Educate patient re discharge instructions and need for follow up.

Source: Alguire P, Whelan G, Rajput V., *The International Medical Graduate's Guide to US Medicine & Residency Training*, Philadelphia, ACP Press; 2009

Readers of previous editions of *Staying Human during Residency Training* and residents who have attended seminars I have given in both Canada and the United States have pointed out that providing endless lists of health risks for trainees seemed discouraging in light of the book's role in emphasizing resident resilience and well-being. I am happy to report that things have improved significantly since the first edition of *Staying Human during Residency Training* came out in 1989!

Here are some key positive trends:

- Residents are now more aware of self-care and are more insistent on achieving balance and resilience in their personal and work lives.
- Work-hour restrictions now exist in both Canada and the United States and continue to be monitored and fine-tuned. New solutions are emerging.[5]
- Most residency programs in North America offer wellness initiatives and resources.
- There has been a significant shift away from a study of physician impairment to looking at physician wellness, humanism, and well-being. A growing literature actually looks at definitions of physician happiness! (More on happiness shortly.)

These are all welcome developments. Nonetheless, residency does present some unique challenges and stressors. Table 1.2 summarizes the top stressors as identified in 1987, 2008, and currently.

Table 1.2 Top Stressors in 1987, 2008, and Nowadays

In 1987:

Insufficient sleep, less than 3 hours
Frequent night calls every third night or more often
Uncompromising attending physicians
Large patient load
Too much scut work
Too much medical records work
High rates of death among patients
Little or no contact with fellow residents
Inadequate sexual activity
High peer competition to impress staff

In 2008:

Work load
Sleep deprivation
Difficult patients
Fear of litigation
Frequent deaths
Information overload
Social isolation
Fear of infection (HIV, SARS, hepatitis)
Dying patients
Lack of personal time

Nowadays:

Time pressures
Finances
The Affordable Healthcare Act, aka Obamacare (in the US)
Medically assisted death (in Canada)
Needle sticks
Abusive, inappropriate house officers
Request to do inappropriate procedures
Competitive classmates
Patient death
Sexual harassment
Difficult violent patients
Difficult family members
Fatigue
Personal family illness
Lack of personal time

Sources: Aminazadeh N, Farrokhyar F, Naeeni M, Reid S, Kashfi A, Kahnamoui K, *Canadian Journal of Surgery* 2012 Aug; 55(4): S145–51.

Although most Canadian and US resident physicians have and maintain a positive outlook, residents still experience significant stressors and a significant proportion may be at risk for emotional and mental health problems. The "Happy Doc" study[6] surveyed residents across all medical schools in Canada and was administered through CAIR, the Canadian Association of Internes and Residents (now called Resident Doctors of Canada). One-third of residents reported their life as "quite a bit to extremely stressful." Time pressure was the most significant factor associated with stress. Intimidation and harassment was experienced by more than half of all residents, most often based on training status (as related to seniority or gender). Eighteen percent of residents reported their mental health as either "fair " or "poor." The two top resources that residents wished to have available were career counseling and financial counseling. These areas have been surprisingly neglected but are now offered in many programs.[7]

Haiku of Residency, by Emily R. Transue

1. Please
Please do not code now;
I have just found a warm spot
in this cold hard bed.

2. Identity
Who am I to you?
White-coated figure folds cold hands,
calls in scripts by phone.

3. Hematemesis
We each have five pints
of blood. I counted your five
in the red basin.

4. Eight A.M.
You say good morning
but does it count as morning
if I did not sleep?

5. Alarm
My pager goes off
Searing explosion of noise
– No, that's a fire drill.

Seven flights of stairs
Run breathless in double steps
My heart fast; yours, still.

RISK CATEGORIES

Here are some sample results of other recent studies on resident health in both Canada and the United States, according to risk categories. These statistics are not meant to be discouraging, but rather serve as a reminder or "ounce of prevention" for you to take good care of yourself and of each other.

IT HAPPENED IN FIRST YEAR
I never liked presenting at Grand Rounds. One false move and you were humiliated.

I was on my cardiac rotation in first year medicine, up on the stage presenting on mitral valve prolapse, when my beeper went off.

I kept talking – only 5 minutes left to go. It went off again.

Then the phone in the auditorium rang. The Chief wanted to speak to me.

I asked them to take a message.

"No, now!," was the answer.

They passed me the portable phone.

I explained I was in the middle of presenting and would call him back right away, but the yelling wouldn't stop.

I had "inadequately diuresed" one of his VIP patients in (cardiac) failure when I was last on call.

I'm pretty sure everyone in the audience heard the tirade word for word.

I blushed. I stuttered. I shook a bit. My body was hunched and deflated. A heart attack of my very own would have been welcome.

> I hung up the phone.
> Nobody said anything.
> I don't even remember presenting my last 3 PowerPoint slides or how I walked down the stairs off the stage.

Burnout, Anxiety, and Depression

- 76% of a sample of first-year internal medicine residents met criteria for burnout.
- 65% of ER residents met criteria for burnout.[8]
- Depression and anxiety symptoms were reported to be 3–4 times more common in a sample of family medicine residents compared with the general public.[9]
- 40% of residents reported impaired performance as a result of anxiety and depression lasting 4 weeks or longer.[10]
- Of a sample of emergency room residents, 30% reported post-traumatic stress disorder symptoms.[11]

Substance Abuse

- 7.6% of 1,555 interns self-prescribed medications.[12]
- A sample of 3,000 third-year residents revealed higher past-month rates of alcohol and benzodiazepam use compared with the general public.[13]

Abuse and Harassment

- 46.4 to 96.5% of medical trainees experienced some form of abuse (verbal, sexual, or physical) during their training.[14]
- Two-thirds of emergency residents worry about their own safety while working shifts.[15]

Suicide

- Physicians under 40 years of age have 3 times the suicide risk of the general population.[16]
- Suicide is the second-greatest cause of death in medical students.[16]

The good news is that residents can be trained to recognize suicide risk in their colleagues.[17,18]

Relationships

- 37–40% of residents report problems with their spouse or lover.[19]
- Of 1,805 residents and interns, 59% believed that role conflict was always or often a problem and that work interfered with their family and social lives.[20]

Job Satisfaction

- Of doctors under age 40 surveyed by the AMA, 31% said they would not have gone to medical school if they had known what they know now.[21]
- A balance between effort and reward is significantly linked to stress (high effort with low reward is a predictor of distress).[22]

Stressors

- Many residents have concerns about job prospects.
- 96% of a sample of obstetrics and gynecology residents were afraid of being sued.[23]
- Training hospitals are being sold, closed, or amalgamated.
- The average resident's salary works out to be less than US $10.00 per hour.
- The average debt load is between $150,000 and $250,000 (see www. amsa.org).
- Although work-hour restrictions have been implemented in the United States and Canada, program non-compliance remains an issue.[24]
- Of graduating residents, 10% feel unprepared for certain clinical challenges, such as substance abuse, domestic violence, geriatrics, and HIV care.

Other Health Risks[25,26]

- IBS
- Hypertension

Table 1.3 Sources of Stress from "Happy Docs" Study

Time pressure, work situation, financial situation, residency program issues, personal relationship, own personal or family responsibilities, own emotional mental health problem, employment status, own physical health problem, caring for own children, caring for others, discrimination, personal family safety

Source: Cohen, Leung, Fahey, et al., The happy docs study – see note 6.

- Infections: needle-stick injuries; hepatitis A, B, C; tuberculosis; SARS; Epstein Barr virus; human immunodeficiency virus – HIV; upper respiratory tract infections; gastroenteritis; conjunctivitis
- Chemical: radiation, anesthetic agents, antineoplastic agents, and agents used in pathology laboratories (e.g., formaldehyde)
- Physical: musculo-skeletal stress related to lifting and prolonged standing, violence from patients, lack of security in hospitals located in dangerous areas
- Athletic deconditioning, weight gain
- Fatigue leading to car accidents post-call, or increased errors on the job
- Increased incidents of pre-term labor and pre-eclampsia among women who become pregnant during residency
- Vitamin D deficiency due to decreased sunlight exposure
- Avoidance of medical care and follow up, perhaps because residents are fearful of being in the patient role

KEY TRENDS AROUND RESIDENCY STRESS

The first year of postgraduate training, especially the first two months on rotations in medicine, surgery, and intensive care units, are frequently reported to be particularly stressful. Studies of working hour reforms suggest that interns (first-year trainees) may have benefitted most from new restrictions.[27] However, senior residents are also reporting high levels of stress related to final examinations, higher expectations, and career planning.[6] Keep in mind that stress-related symptoms are ubiquitous and intermittent, even when they do not become severe enough to lead to depression or drug abuse. As you'll see, resilience in the face of stress can be learned and maintained. Prolonged symptoms can, however, lead to professional burnout, which is characterized by emotional exhaustion, depersonalization, detachment, and a low sense of personal accomplishment and job satisfaction.[22] Burnout is defined as a deteriorating or unsuccessful response to repeated stress and is characterized by negative attitude toward oneself, others, and work, emotional exhaustion, and feelings of despair. It leads to what Maslach calls erosion of the soul. (Other authors have referred to "training toxicity" as being the cause of such stress.[28] For excellent reviews on burnout in medical residents, see Prins,[29] Niku,[30] and McCray.[31])

So, are you burnt out? Ask yourself the predictive questions from the Maslach inventory shown here. Keep in mind that when you take the test (post-call vs while on holiday) will determine your score!

Modified Questions from Maslach Burnout Inventory:[32]

Depersonalization:
1 I feel I treat some patients as if they were impersonal objects.
2 I do not really care what happens to some patients.
3 Patients blame me for some of their problems.

Emotional exhaustion:
1 I still feel tired when I wake up on workday mornings.

Personal accomplishment:
1 I can easily understand how my patients feel about things.
2 I deal effectively with my patients' problems.
3 I can easily create a relaxed atmosphere for my patients.
4 I feel exhilarated after working closely with my patients.

MAJOR MANIFESTATIONS OF BURNOUT[33]

Physiological

Fatigue and chronic exhaustion, recurrent upper respiratory tract infections, persistent viral infections, headaches, lack of concentration, somatic problems, muscular pain and tension, weight problems, gastrointestinal disorders, and injuries caused by high-risk behavior are all physiological manifestations of burnout.

Psychological and Emotional

Negative thoughts and feelings (despair, feelings of impotence, boredom, disillusionment, guilt, reduced self-esteem, irritability, social isolation) are major psychological and emotional manifestations of burnout.

Behavioral

Shutting down emotionally, absenteeism, unproductivity, hyperactivity, exaggerated response to stress, inappropriate comments, social withdrawal, increased risk taking). Some residents experience these symptoms only during a particularly difficult rotation. However, others experience full-blown burnout and what has been called "the house officer's stress syndrome," which is characterized by family problems, cynical attitudes, emotional lability and anger, personal conflict, and transient cognitive impairment. One study of internal-medicine residents using the Maslach Burnout Inventory showed that 76% of respondents met the criteria for burnout.[34]

It's no surprise that the number of hours worked per week appears to be the best predictor of professional burnout. Apart from somatic and emotional symptoms, high levels of chronic malaise in young physicians can produce a lasting change of attitude toward both the medical field and patients. Residency can be a time for learning coping patterns for an active, demanding medical career and for attaining new levels of compassion and resilience. However, as you've probably already noticed, some graduates emerge as insensitive, distant, cynical, and authoritarian physicians who make inappropriate comments and judgments about their patients. They become emotionally withdrawn and self-important and their self-esteem becomes intrinsically linked to, or exclusively defined by, professional and financial performance to the neglect of satisfying personal relationships. When several members of the healthcare team are experiencing burnout, an organizational impact is noted as well. There is a decline in quality of services and a toxic climate of hostility, competition, and mistrust develops. There are authority conflicts and impaired communications, leading to decision making in isolation.

Summary

The 3 Faces of Burnout: Exhaustion, Cynicism, Inefficiency

INDIVIDUAL VULNERABILITIES

We all have our own personality traits, strengths, and quirks, shaped by genetics and our early family lives. The literature on resident impairment allows some degree of prediction about who among us may be at risk in the face of high stress levels. An editorial in the *Annals of Internal Medicine* even posed the question "Who is sicker, patients or residents?"[35] Residents who over-identify with patients and have passive-aggressive, avoidant, or dependent coping styles are predisposed to burnout. Those having difficulty expressing difficult emotions also struggle (i.e., those with an obsessive personality style). Hostile or aggressive type A residents may alienate their colleagues. Those who lack support from colleagues, friends, and families exhibit more symptoms of somatic and psychological origin and are more detached and avoidant. Trainees who can't delegate responsibility or share teamwork also become more stressed.[36]

Most residents occasionally experience feelings of loss of control over their lives and even over decisions about patient care. Those who reported "an external locus of control" (where others make decisions for them) also have higher stress levels. Certain psychological defense mechanisms that we all have to some degree can also lead to difficulties. These include denial and rationalization about failures, errors, and limitations, deprecation (ironic or disrespectful humor), isolation of affect (emotional numbness or dissociation), and projection of negative feelings onto others. Many residents believe that they don't learn to communicate effectively with patients during their training, so burdened are they by technology, medical jargon, and the safe anonymity of group work and laboratory-result rounding. Time pressures, fatigue, and maintaining self-confidence tend to be the focus of the most difficult or stressful aspects of residency training. Other sources of stress, apart from those listed in table 1.2, include role ambiguity with expectations beyond one's level of expertise, ethical dilemmas, time management struggles, lack of mentoring or role models, and conflicts in personal and professional relationships. Read on for tips on coping with all of these.

Generational clashes with older physicians who doubt the dedication of a new breed of "balance minded trainees" (especially in the context of recent work-hour regulations) are increasingly common. Older doctors have often defined their lives by service, availability, and sacrifice, while younger physicians are more aware of the need to take good care of themselves in order to take care of patients and to sustain efficacy over time. These are very different worldviews and a middle ground needs to be found and discussed openly.

DEVELOPMENTAL ISSUES

Most residents in North America are 25 to 30 years old. In the most frequently studied groups – psychiatry, internal medicine, and family medicine programs – those in their early twenties and late thirties seem to be more affected by the rigors of residency.[37] One study showed that women housestaff experienced more self-doubt and feelings of professional inadequacy.[37]

Trends in difficulties delegating duties for women have also been noted (see chapter 7). Family practice residents have worried most about making mistakes in treatment and diagnosis and residents in psychiatry were most concerned about chronically ill patients. On-call anxiety was more frequent among residents in family medicine, psychiatry, and pediatrics.[38] It's hard to have to prove yourself over and over on new rotations. The particular challenges experienced by specific resident groups, including women and international medical graduates, are discussed in chapter 7.

If you're not careful, the professional stresses of residency may adversely affect or postpone personal development and key milestones because of a lack of time to reflect and explore creatively. Young physicians in their twenties and thirties customarily leave their families in home towns, and experience changes in financial status. They date, form sexual relationships, marry or cohabit, and have children. Many women physicians postpone having children despite fertility rates falling over time. Some residents divorce, become ill, or experience a loss in their families. They search for a balance between work and play and develop interests in political and community causes.

WHAT RESIDENTS WANT[39]

A Canadian study based on surveying respondents from several provincial housestaff organizations led to a report called "Features of High Quality Residency Programs – A National Resident Perspective" (http://residentdoctors.ca). The following components of an ideal program were identified:

- A collegial working environment free from intimidation and harassment
- Adequate transition to practice, preparation including appropriate, graded responsibility over time
- An appropriate education to maintain a balance of life and service
- Mentorship from the program director and faculty supervisor
- A curriculum with diverse clinical and procedure exposures
- Timely assessments with face-to-face feedback
- A program director who is supportive of resident concerns

It's indeed encouraging that residents are increasingly able to identify what they need to thrive, and then be willing to request it from their program directors. They are also familiar with a growing literature emphasizing resident wellness rather than the previous focus on risk and impairment. Some of the predictors of increased personal growth during residency include:[40] setting a time for reflection; having a strong desire to develop personally as well as professionally; maintaining a strong sense of self; feeling committed to core personal values; and feeling supported in one's life. Furthermore, although some educators disagree, a number of studies have looked at and confirmed the health-related and professional benefits of reduced work hours in North American residency programs.[41] Emerging evidence[41] suggests that the development of the following skills is associated with improved personal health outcomes and professional sustainability:

1 Personal awareness: being aware of values, beliefs, assumptions, and worldview, having a reflective practice.
2 Critical appraisal of the self, which includes introspection: this means being able to look at a specific situation, describe it, identify feelings about what happened, then look at what went well, what didn't go well, form conclusions, and make an action plan for change. At the University of Toronto, we also emphasize specific ways of thinking and being:
   (a) Narrative competence (the ability to work empathically with stories)
   (b) Critical analysis (the ability to question where knowledge comes from)

(c) Visual literacy (the ability to work with non-verbal cues)
Read on for more information on these attributes.

3 Emotional intelligence: the ability to perceive, understand, and manage emotions in one's self and others. A recent study showed that emotional intelligence can, in part, be taught and that emotional quotient (EQ) scores can actually increase significantly over the course of training![42] You can check your EQ at www.queendom.com and www.greatergood.berkeley.edu/ei_quiz. For tips on being an emotionally intelligent team member, see p. 95.

4 Leadership: As you've observed, the contemporary doctor plays a complex role in the process of ensuring the community's health. Doctors are expected to be leaders in their communities and in their clinical setting, to be articulate, to advocate for their patients, to have a clear sense of their own values and beliefs, and to have the skills to attract and maintain relationships with others in a way that motivates action based on integrity.

TIP: *"I have benefited enormously from keeping a little log of my experiences. I think a lot of residents can benefit from keeping a diary. I am careful never to mention anyone by name, it is a private thing, it is never to be published, but it's nice to look back on who I was."*

5 Well-being, resilience, and happiness: the formation of a sound professional and work identity as a physician cannot be achieved independently of other developmental concerns, although the latter are sometimes ignored. Young physicians must be able to find a balance between their own vulnerability and their role as non-omnipotent healers.[34] You must recognize when to act and when to wait, observe, and listen. Residents sometimes feel helpless and exploited in the medical hierarchy, but must develop problem-solving skills, assertiveness, and expertise in order to allow feelings of commitment to develop with a regained sense of personal control. You must learn boundary maintenance, combining empathy with objectivity, and avoiding both undue familiarity and aloofness with colleagues and patients. Residents can and should acquire these skills and insights during their residency training. The emerging healer must

Figure 1.1 Stress and Coping Model for Physicians

Source: May, HH, Revicki, DA, 'Professional Stress among Family Physicians,' *J Fam Pract* 1985; 20: 165–71.

develop a sense of identity, balance, and well-being in the face of professional and developmental stressors. The potential risks to both physical and emotional health may be significant, but so are the opportunities to learn resilience and coping skills that will last throughout your life and medical career.

Figure 1.1 offers one model of successful versus unsuccessful coping.

It's a useful exercise for you to define what well-being means to you as a doctor. The following list provides a "definition"[43] that includes the key elements of that state.

Elements of Physician Well-being[39,44]

- Quality care, including continuity of care
- Commitment to professional values and professional growth
- Shared responsibility with the patient for the patient's health and well-being
- Full expression of the physician as an autonomous person
- Maintenance of personal, physical, and mental health
- Balance of family, social, physical, mental, spiritual, creative, and financial domains
- Self-validation and personal satisfaction
- Recognition and acceptance of time and technological limitations, of change as a normal phenomenon, and of the profession's inherent problems and opportunities
- Collegiality, teamwork, and work group loyalty, i.e., a sense of belonging.

RESILIENCE

The flip side to burnout is definitely resilience. Resilient physicians have increased career satisfaction, higher personal life satisfaction, enhanced performance and efficacy, and an engagement with life-long learning and skills.

Resilience can be defined as a process of adapting well in the face of stress, trauma, adversity, tragedy, or threat. Resilience does not mean that you never get stressed. It means being able to bounce back from difficult experiences and to learn from them.

Other factors associated with resilience include having caring and supportive relationships, being able to make realistic plans and taking steps to carry them out. Having a positive view of oneself, being able to communicate and problem solve, and having the capacity to manage strong feelings and impulses are also key aspects. A common misconception is that some people have "grit" and others do not.

The American Psychological Association identifies the following 10 ways to build resilience:

1 Make connections.
2 Avoid seeing crises as insurmountable problems.
3 Accept change as a part of living. (One piece of graffiti I once read said, CHANGE IS INEVITABLE. GROWTH IS OPTIONAL.)
4 Move toward realistic goals.
5 Take decisive actions.
6 Look for opportunities for self-discovery.
7 Nurture a positive view of yourself, including self-confidence.
8 Keep things in perspective, and don't blow them out of proportion.
9 Maintain a hopeful outlook.
10 Take care of yourself with proper diet, exercise, and sleep (see chapter 3).

(Adapted from: www.apa.org)

For physicians, the following elements are also highly predictive of professional resilience:

1 A sense of self and personal competence and agency, as well as possessing personal beliefs
2 Attitudes and perspective also correlate with being self-aware, reflective, and attuned, having core values and an optimistic philosophy of life, and being ultra-realistic
3 Having a healthy temperament and a sense of humor; not taking things personally
4 Acceptance of self and others, and being able to forgive self and others
5 Feeling that one is making a difference in one's profession (purpose)
6 An ability to learn from past challenges and stressful situations

For an example of a superb resilience curriculum, go to the Dartmouth Geisel Resilience web page: http://sites.dartmouth.edu/Geisel-resilience-curriculum-resources/.

WHAT ABOUT HAPPINESS?

It is encouraging that nowadays we are not only speaking about physician well-being, but about what defines happiness for all human beings, including physicians. As mentioned above, we all start with genetic strengths and vulnerabilities and our personalities are shaped by our early family experiences. Predictors of quality of life in residency include satisfaction with the program, seniority (year 2 and 3), time for leisure, and less than 30 hours per week of caring for critically ill patients.[45]

Happier residents have reported improved relationships with patients and colleagues, improved patient care, and greater motivation ("zeal") for their work.[46] Martin Seligman[47] and others have looked at the science of happiness and what features determine it. Interestingly, they found that this has nothing to do with climate, wealth, or the number of years of education. (This may be important because some residents tell themselves that these things will make them happy.) It's all about the 2 P's: having a sense of purpose and pleasure in your life. Here are actual predictors of happiness based on Seligman's research:

- Finding meaning in one's work
- Not dwelling on negative events, errors, or self-criticism (i.e., an optimistic outlook)
- Being part of a couple and having a strong social network, which includes family relationships
- Financial stability but not excessive wealth
- Good health
- Personal freedom and the opportunity to live by one's personal values

Other important ingredients identified by Seligman include developing a sense of day-to-day gratitude and seeking/offering forgiveness.

The chapters that follow will provide concrete strategies aimed not only at coping, but at finding the potential for happiness in your complex role as an apprentice physician. This means paying close attention to your unique personal development, to mental and physical health, to relationships, and to developing an authentic sense of self with values you can live by. The overall residency training system has improved, but it's not perfect. You can learn to manage your stress and become the kind of healer (and human being) you want to be!

REFERENCES

1 Graduate medical education, Appendix II, Table 1. *JAMA*. 1996;276(9):739–48. http://dx.doi.org/10.1001/jama.1996.03540090085019.

2 CAPER annual census of post-M.D. trainees, 1996–1997. Association of Canadian Medical Colleges, Ottawa, 1997.

3 Blachly PH, Osterud HT, Josslin R. Suicide in professional groups. *N Engl J Med*. 1963;268(23):1278–82. http://dx.doi.org/10.1056/NEJM196306062682307.

4 McCue JD. The effects of stress on physicians and their medical practice. *N Engl J Med*. 1982;306(8):458–63. http://dx.doi.org/10.1056/NEJM198202253060805.

5 Pattani R, Wu P, Irfan A, Dhalla IA. Resident duty hours in Canada: Past, present and future. *CMAJ*. 2014;186(10):761–5. http://dx.doi.org/10.1503/cmaj.131053.

6 Cohen JS, Leung Y, Fahey M, et al. The happy docs study: A Canadian Association of Internes and Residents well-being survey examining resident physician health and satisfaction within and outside of residency training in Canada. *BMC Res Notes*. 2008;1(1):105. http://dx.doi.org/10.1186/1756-0500-1-105.

7 Block L, Wu AW, Feldman L, et al. Residency schedule, burnout and patient care among first-year residents. *Postgrad Med J*. 2013;89(1055):495–500. http://dx.doi.org/10.1136/postgradmedj-2012-131743.

8 Takayesu JK, Ramoska EA, Clark TR, et al. Factors associated with burnout during emergency medicine residency. *JAEM*. 2014;9(21):1031–5.

9 Kelly EL. Coping strategies, depression and anxiety among Ontario family medicine residents. *Can Fam Physician*. 2005;51:242–3.

10 Koran L, Litt I. House staff well-being. *West J Med*. 1988;148:97–401.

11 Mills LD, Mills TJ. Symptoms of post-traumatic stress disorder among emergency medicine residents. *J Emerg Med*. 2005;28(1):1–4. http://dx.doi.org/10.1016/j.jemermed.2004.05.009.

12 Guille C, Sen S. Prescription drug use and self-prescription among trained physicians. *Arch Intern Med*. 2012;172(4):371–2. http://dx.doi.org/10.1001/archinternmed.2011.791.

13 Hughes PH, Conrad SE, Baldwin DC. Resident physician substance use in the United States. *JAMA*. 1991;265:2069–73. http://dx.doi.org/10.1001/jama.1991.03460160047027.

14 Silver HK, Slicken A. Medical student abuse: Incidence, severity and significance. *JAMA*. 1990;263(4):527–32. http://dx.doi.org/10.1001/jama.1990.03440040066030.

15 Anglin D, Kyriacou DN, Hutson HR. Residents' perspectives on violence and personal safety in the emergency department. *Ann Emerg Med.* 1994;23(5):1082–4. http://dx.doi.org/10.1016/S0196-0644(94)70108-3.

16 Ross M. Suicide among physicians. *Psychiatry Med.* 1971;2(3):189–98. http://dx.doi.org/10.2190/0DUY-Y1LX-EQNY-4J8L.

17 Hochberg MS, Berman RS, Kalet AL, et al. The stress of residency: recognizing the signs of depression and suicide in you and your fellow residents. *Am J Surg.* 2013;205(2):141–6. http://dx.doi.org/10.1016/j.amjsurg.2012.08.003.

18 Knight JM. Physiological and neurobiological aspects of stress and their relevance for residency training. *Acad Psychiatry.* 2013;37(1):6–10. http://dx.doi.org/10.1176/appi.ap.11100187.

19 Landau C, Hall S, Wartman SA, et al. Stress in social and family relationships during medical residency. *J Med Educ.* 1986;61:654–60.

20 PAIRO study. www.pairo.org.

21 Reported in *Globe and Mail Report on Business.* June 1994. See also www.ama-assn.org.

22 Sakata Y, Wada K, Tsutsumi A, et al. Effort-reward imbalance and depression in Japanese medical residents. *J Occup Health.* 2008;50(6):498–504. http://dx.doi.org/10.1539/joh.L8043.

23 Carius M. Avoiding "training toxicity" staying human during residency. *Ann Emerg Med.* 2001;38(5):596–7. http://dx.doi.org/10.1067/mem.2001.119425.

24 Madsen T. A long wait for shorter shifts. *The New Physician* 2009. http://www.amsa.org/404.

25 Wells MM, Roth L, Chande N. Sleep disruption secondary to overnight call shifts is associated with irritable bowel syndrome in residents: A cross-sectional study. *Am J Gastroenterol.* 2012;107(8):1151–6. http://dx.doi.org/10.1038/ajg.2011.486.

26 Gupta HO, Gupta S, Carter RL, et al. Does orthopaedic surgical training induce hypertension? A pilot study. *Clin Orthop Relat Res.* 2012;470(11):3253–60. http://dx.doi.org/10.1007/s11999-012-2491-4.

27 Drolet BC, Christopher DA, Fischer SA. Residents' response to duty-hour regulations – a follow-up national survey. *N Engl J Med.* 2012;366(24):e35. http://dx.doi.org/10.1056/NEJMp1202848.

28 Hyman SA, Michaels DR, Berry JM, et al. Risk of burnout in perioperative clinicians. *Anesthesiology.* 2011;114(1):194–204. http://dx.doi.org/10.1097/ALN.0b013e318201ce9a.

29 Prins JT, Gazendam-Donofrio SM, Tubben BJ, et al. Burnout in medical residents: A review. *Med Educ.* 2007;41(8):788–800. http://dx.doi.org/10.1111/j.1365-2923.2007.02797.x.

30 Niku T. Resident burnout. *JAMA*. 2004;292:2888–9.

31 McCray LW, Cronholm PF, Bogner HR, et al. Resident burnout: Is there hope? *Fam Med*. 2008;40(9):626–32.

32 Bouchard F, Bélanger P, editors. *Putting the Heat on Burnout, Health and Safety*. Committee of the Fédération des infirmières et infirmiers de Québec. Quebec: Litho Acme; 1989.

33 Shanafelt TD, Bradley KA, Wipf JE, et al. Burnout and self-reported patient care in an internal medicine residency program. *Ann Intern Med*. 2002;136(5):358–67. http://dx.doi.org/10.7326/0003-4819-136-5-200203050-00008.

34 Hawes L. Who is sicker: Patients or residents? Residents' distress and the care of patients. *Ann Intern Med*. 2002;136(5):391–3. http://dx.doi.org/10.7326/0003-4819-136-5-200203050-00012.

35 Mazie B. Job stress, psychological health, and social support of family practice residents. *J Med Educ*. 1985;60:935–41.

36 Rudner HL. Work-related stress: A survey of family practice residents in Ontario. *Can Fam Physician*. 1988;34:577–83.

37 Russell AT, Pasnace RO, Taintor ZC. Emotional problems of residents in psychiatry. *Am J Psychiatry*. 1975;132(3):263–7. http://dx.doi.org/10.1176/ajp.132.3.263.

38 Vogel L. Just a little respect, please. *CMAJ*. 2011;183(8):895. http://dx.doi.org/10.1503/cmaj.109-3850.

39 Wright S, Levine RB, Beasley B, et al. Personal growth and its correlates during residency training. *Med Educ*. 2006;40(8):737–45. http://dx.doi.org/10.1111/j.1365-2929.2006.02499.x.

40 Fletcher KE, Underwood W III, Davis SQ, et al. Effects of work hour reduction on residents' lives: A systematic review. *JAMA*. 2005;294(9):1088–100. http://dx.doi.org/10.1001/jama.294.9.1088.

41 Puddester D, Flynn L, Cohen J, eds. *CanMEDS Physician Health Guide: A Practical Handbook for Physician Health and Well-being*. Royal College of Physicians and Surgeons of Canada; e-book available at www.royalcollege.ca/canmeds (the Royal College of Physicians and Surgeons of Canada CANMEDS Physician Health Guide, adapted with permission).

42 Satterfield J, Swenson S, Rabow M. Emotional intelligence in internal medicine residents: Educational implications for clinical performance and burnout. *Ann Behav Sci Med Educ*. 2009;14(2):65–8.

43 Dyrbye LN, Satele D, Sloan J, et al. Utility of a brief screening tool to identify physicians in distress. *J Gen Intern Med*. 2012;28:421–7. http://dx.doi.org/10.1007/s11606-012-2252-9.

44 Brent DA. The residency as a developmental process. *J Med Educ*. 1981;56:417–22.

45 Macedo PCM, Citero V, Schenkman S, et al. Health-related quality of life predictors during medical residency in a random, stratified sample of residents. *Rev Bras Psiquiatr.* 2009;31(2):119–24. http://dx.doi.org/10.1590/S1516-44462009000200007.

46 Ratanawongsa N, Wright S, Carrese JA. Well-being in residency: Effects on relationships with patients, interactions with colleagues, performance and motivation. *Patient Educ Couns.* 2008;72(2):194–200. http://dx.doi.org/10.1016/j.pec.2008.04.010. ·

47 Seligman M. *Authentic Happiness: Using the New Positive Psychology to Realize Your Potential for Lasting Fulfillment.* New York: Free Press; 2003.

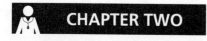

CHAPTER TWO

Preventive Medicine:
Choosing a Humane Residency

In the past, graduating medical students, when choosing a residency program in North America, focused more on the program's reputed standards or prestige than on the quality of life they could expect during that 4- to 6-year period of their lives. They sometimes based their choices on hearsay or on information acquired by chance. In interviews they concentrated on practical questions such as the size of a program or the opportunities it offered for research. Because selection was highly competitive, students seldom introduced other, more humanistic concerns for fear of appearing demanding or not sufficiently dedicated. Nowadays, medical students are figuring lifestyle choices and balance into their choice of specialty, and they are receiving guidance in career choices. And, it's about time!

Two trends in North America seem to have produced a change in the attitudes of candidates and residency directors toward such concerns. First, the growing number of women in medicine, who now constitute 50% or more of most US and Canadian medical classes, has forced universities to consider part-time and shared residencies as well as parental leaves. Such modifications in response to women's demands have been achieved with great struggle; yet men now acknowledge that they also benefit from these new policies.[1]

Second, restrictions on the number of hours worked by interns and residents in Canada (which was a pioneer in this regard), the United States, and the European Union have thankfully legitimized discussions of resident health, lifestyle, and well-being worldwide.

Residency training programs have thus become more sensitive to residents' growth and comfort than was the case 10 years ago. Overall, the choice of program has become more complicated because more factors now influence the selection of a specialty and training programs. Navigating the Match is an art in and of itself! (See the additional resources on applying for residency and tips on the match in chapter 13 for more information.)

SPECIALTY CHOICE

Program Factors

Because of the considerable variation in the size, content, and administration of residency programs across the United States and Canada, medical graduates must exercise great care in their choice of program to try to ensure maximum learning and personal satisfaction.[2] This means gathering a large body of information about each center from a variety of sources before applying, because it is not possible to discover accurately all the features of a program in a single interview.

Data should be obtained from the program or hospital prospectus, medical school counselors, and published specialty manuals such as the Fellowship and Residency Electronic Interactive Database (FREIDA), the National Resident Matching Program Handbook for Students (see Resources) and, in Canada, the Canadian Resident Matching Service (www.carms.ca). Local faculty members at the undergraduate and postgraduate levels and student members of specialty associations (who often link up on Facebook and via blogs) can also be sources of information.

Classmates gathering similar data can share facts and ideas. It's a good idea to make informal contact with junior and senior residents at each center being considered, or perhaps with graduates of one's own school, and to obtain a copy of the hospital, provincial, or state contract for residents. Observerships during clerkship are helpful. Doing an elective there during med school is also a good idea, but experiences may vary considerably from site to site. A day-long visit to the teaching hospital can help one assess working conditions and resident morale.

Applicants should ensure that they have gathered all pertinent information before accepting a residency position.

Here are key considerations most residents take into account when selecting a specialty:[3]

- Spousal preference regarding lifestyle and location (though climate does not actually impact stress levels!)
- Lifestyle and workload
- Job and academic prospects
- Competitiveness and availability of programs
- Expected salary and medical school debt load
- Lawsuit potential
- Sexual stereotyping
- Age preference (young vs old patients)
- Length of training
- Balance between emphasis on patient contact and communication skills and on manual and technical skills
- Research potential, scientific interests
- Local licensing requirements ("portability" of the specialty)
- Personal issues (family or personal history of a particular illness or exposure to specific specialty care)
- Success and satisfaction levels in undergraduate rotations
- Positive exposure to resident or mentor role models
- Family factors (family member in the same specialty, partner's preferences)
- Intellectual preference and background
- Availability of subspecialty options
- Personality style
- Public and media perceptions of the specialty
- Perceived personal health risk (burnout, infectious diseases)
- Government manpower "shortage" policies (incentives and disincentives) affecting practice-setting options on graduation
- Autonomy versus team approach
- Debt load (Sadly, many trainees in the United States still avoid family medicine, a career they would enjoy, because of financial constraints. In contrast, family medicine is a popular choice in Canada.)
- Job prospects (Physician unemployment actually happens.)

Picking a Specialty

Here are some great career counseling websites that will help you decide which specialty fits your talents, personality, and learning style:

Careers in Medicine: https://www.aamc.org/cim/
Medical Specialty Aptitude Test: http://www.med-ed.virginia.edu/
  Specialties/

CONSIDERATIONS IN CHOOSING A RESIDENCY[3]

Here are some factors to contemplate as you make your decision.

The Program

- Accreditation data and ratings
- Number of residents in each year of the program and the number expected to begin in the first year of the next session
- Compliance with work-hour restrictions
- Number of hospitals in the program
- Union/housestaff association resources
- Amount of time spent in each hospital
- Financial resources of the program
- Location of each hospital
- Amount, location, and flexibility in scheduling and content of elective time
- Amount of supervision, volume of activity, and length of shifts in emergency rotations
- Anticipated major changes in program policy or administration that might affect residents
- Availability of rural primary-care rotations and clinical exposure
- Area housing/schools
- Cost of living in the specific urban center
- Potential for advancement (postgraduate – MA/PhD programs – fellowships, chief residency, and staff positions)
- Availability of job-sharing options
- Success rate of residents in fellowship or board exams
- Availability of support groups and residency well-being resources (see chapter 4)

- Resident satisfaction/input to program design
- Policies on diversity/equity
- Disability accommodations
- Availability of intimidation/harassment policies
- Availability of concurrent graduate degree training (i.e., ethics/ humanity, etc.) and combined residency (i.e., med-peds, pedspsych, FM-ER)
- Gut feeling (don't discount this!)

The Institution

- Unionized or nonunionized; availability of resident representation or collective bargaining (Some programs don't like the word "union," so look for availability of contracts/collective agreements.)
- Type (specialized, military, veterans, private, county, provincial, or state)
- Availability of resources and innovative techniques
- Number of beds and admissions per year
- Research and teaching possibilities
- Friendly to international medical graduates (IMGs)
- Friendly to cultural, religious, and sexual minorities
- Popularity of the hospital among housestaff
- Commitment to teaching versus service
- Involvement of HMOs or managed care and how that affects exposure to a broad clinical base and continuity of care
- Patient type (geographical area served, socioeconomic and ethnic status, variety in age, and proportion of acute vs chronic problems)
- Commitment to resident well-being
- Community vs hospital-based

Attending Staff

- Background of the service chief, department head, chief resident, and attending staff
- Availability of the residency training director
- Interest and availability of staff for teaching, consulting, supervising, and mentoring

- Exposure to well-known clinicians in the field
- Emphasis on innovation
- Supportive attitudes to team members

Duties

- Time spent on service versus teaching
- Expected ward patient load
- Organization of rotations: emergency, elective, chronic, clinic, and inpatient
- Frequency of night calls, number of residents on call, and extent of cross-coverage of wards
- Scheduling of rounds (mornings, weekends, etc.)
- Expectations regarding follow-up on patients treated on wards or in emergency department
- "Scut" level and availability of support staff: nurses, physicians' assistants and extenders, paramedics, blood and intravenous drip teams, messengers, porters, librarians, secretarial staff, and medical records staff
- Record of compliance with legislated limits to number of hours worked and contract protections
- Types of electronic medical records employed

THE HUMAN FACTOR[4]

Learning and training considerations should always be balanced against those that affect your desired quality of life. Residents pay rent, manage debts, go on holiday, have social commitments, and perhaps raise a family. Therefore, you'll need financial information on salary level, frequency of payment (weekly or biweekly), and possibly options for moonlighting. Benefits such as life, health, disability, and malpractice insurance should be provided or made available at reasonable rates through the hospital housestaff union or local medical association. Find out what you can from senior residents in the program.

You may want to know about policies and practices on maternity or paternity leave, job sharing, part-time residency, and compassionate and sick leave. Are wellness resources available (e.g., mentoring, tutoring, fitness facilities, personal counseling)? The size of the program will determine the level of familiarity and intimacy among staff, residents, and patients. Some trainees may view residency as a time to explore new approaches and lifestyles in a new city; others may decide to settle where they have completed medical school so as to build a reputation and career there.

Applicants also need to learn about the availability, cost, and safety of housing, and about its proximity to the hospital. They may want to know whether schools, day care, and shopping facilities are nearby. A support system of family and friends provides protection against stress during residency, and its presence or absence may affect the decision to relocate. Climate and cultural events or athletic facilities may also be important considerations.

Some residents believe that raising such matters during an interview may jeopardize their chances of acceptance because they may introduce personal information – about marital status, sexual orientation, plans to have children, health, and so on – that may not be supplied otherwise. It may be wise to obtain information about these issues elsewhere, but a program that penalizes an applicant for raising them, or that has no provision for such benefits or resources, may not be the one for you.

This personal and professional information must be sorted out if applicants are to choose a program where they will learn happily. Family members, medical school counselors or mentors, friends, and significant others should all be recruited to help weigh the elements involved. For a wonderful resource on coping as a couple and family, written by a medical spouse, see *Surviving Residency* by Kristen Math.

THE INTERVIEW

This is your chance to determine if a program is right for you. Dress professionally and comfortably, and pay attention to grooming. Arm yourself with as much information as possible about a program before your interview. You can then be attentive to important details that will help you make your final decision. Was the program helpful and flexible in making arrangements to meet you? Were interviewers punctual? Did they refer to your CV and ask pertinent questions related to it? Did they put you at ease? (One resident in psychiatry reported some years back that an interviewer, believe it or not, asked him to leave the room and return as his mother!) Know and note the names and titles or positions of all interviewers and consider sending them a follow-up thank-you note. Be courteous to all support staff you contact around the interviews because it's the right thing to do, and they may be asked their opinion of you. Certain topics and questions should not be raised by interviewers in Canada and the United States because they are inappropriate on human rights grounds. You should nevertheless prepare for them because they invariably arise.

THE INTERVIEW

I'd been to enough interviews already that I was almost ready to sleepwalk through the questions I expected: "Why do you want to pursue this specialty? What attracts you to our program?" I knew my interviewers and was sure about how they'd interact with me. I was paired with a good cop and a bad cop: a friendly resident I'd worked with before, and the head of the program, a thin, severe woman who never wasted her time on a smile. At least, that was what I thought until they opened their mouths. And then the questions started.

"So," said the resident, looking wounded, "most of your personal statement is about how much you love another specialty. Are you actually interested in our program?"

It took almost a minute for me to think the unthinkable thought: I really had submitted the wrong personal statement to the program. Every answer I gave turned into an apology. No, I tried to say, I really did love their program. I really wanted to be in it. But the damage was done. In their eyes, it seemed, any attempts to repair the damage meant that I was sloppy at best and a liar at worst.

There was a second interview an hour later, with another interviewer I'd also worked with. In between, I scrambled to find a computer and print off the personal statement I'd meant to send. The second interviewer was another staff physician

I'd worked with. I figured I might as well start by addressing my mistake.

"I submitted the wrong personal statement," I said. "Here's the one I actually meant to submit."

His usual broad smile burst into a laugh. "Don't worry about it," he said. "These things happen. I know you want this specialty. Let's talk about your research experience and what we can offer."

Inappropriate Interview Questions

Here are some examples of inappropriate interview questions:

- How old are you?
- What is your marital status?
- What is your sexual orientation?
- What is your nationality/ citizenship?
- Do you have plans for marriage or pregnancy?
- Outline your medical and psychiatric history.
- What is your HIV sero-status?
- Have you had drug/alcohol problems?
- What is your ethnic, religious, and family background?
- Will you select the program if you are ranked highly? (This violates match agreements, though you may wish to volunteer this information. Don't rely on verbal promises.)
- Where else have you interviewed?

Asking "May I know why you ask that?" in response to such questions suggests to the interviewer that certain details are private and gives you time to compose a suitable response.

Some provocative questions are reasonable and appropriate. You should not only expect them but also rehearse your replies, because they will give an interviewer an accurate sense of your character and career goals. Be sure to appear interested, motivated, and enthusiastic.

Expected Interview Questions

Here are some examples of questions that you should expect during an interview:

- Tell me about yourself. What makes you unique?
- What are your weaknesses and strengths?
- What are your long-term plans?
- Is there anything about you that might prevent you from successfully completing your residency in "x" years?
- What is your most important achievement to date?
- Why have you selected "x" as a specialty? Why not "y"?
- What is the most significant error you have made in your clinical work so far? How did you correct it?
- What attracted you to this program?
- What are your interests outside of medicine?
- Have you any questions about our program?
- Tell me about an interesting/memorable patient.
- What would you change in our healthcare system?
- Have you any plans to do research or teach?
- What does it mean to be professional?
- How are you at teamwork?
- Where do you plan to be 10 years from now?
- What do you want out of life?
- Tell me about a significant medical error you witnessed an how you dealt with it.
- Tell me about "x" (a recent news event or recent medical breakthrough).
- What have you been reading outside of medicine lately?

Residency interviews go both ways. It's fair for you to make certain inquiries as well. The following are some questions you should ask faculty:[4]

- What makes this program unique?
- Why did you train here and stay on?
- What are the strengths, innovations, and weaknesses of the program?

- What is resident morale like? How family-friendly is the program?
- Are any major changes pending?
- Where do most of your graduates go/work?

You might also pose questions for residents at the program:[5]

- What's call like?
- What do you like/dislike about the program? What is the quality o teaching and supervision?
- What made you choose this program? Are you glad you did?
- What resources/well-being/social programs are in place for residents?

PREPARING A CURRICULUM VITAE

A professional-looking CV can move you up to the top of the interview pile. Here are some suggestions for preparing one. Print the following clearly on quality white 8½ x 11 inch paper.

Sample Curriculum Vitae Outline –
DATE IT, check for typos, and send a clean, typed copy!

Personal Information:
- Full name
- Citizenship
- Languages (optional)
- Home address, telephone number, email address
- Professional address, telephone number, email address
- Present academic rank and position (if applicable)

Education:
- Name of institution, degree(s), and date(s)
- College/University
- Medical school
- Residency
- Fellowship
- Other

Certification (i.e., CMCC, USMLE):
- Certificate number

Board Certification (if applicable):
• List month and year of successful completion

Medical Licensure (if applicable):
• Indicate province/state and license number only

Honors and Awards (including scholarships):
• List chronologically, beginning with earliest appointment

Military or Volunteer Service (if applicable):
• List branch of service, rank, place and dates

Academic Appointments and Positions:
• Example: Academic research, clinical appointments
• List chronologically, beginning with earliest appointment Teaching:
• List dates and names of courses taught, time spent as leader of rounds, seminars presented, student advisor roles filled, etc.
• Medical school
• Graduate school
• Continuing education
• Other institutions
• Other relevant past employment

Journals:
• List membership on editorial boards, positions as scientific reviewer for medical journals, etc.
• List chronologically, beginning with earliest appointment

Institutional, Departmental and Divisional Administrative Responsibilities, Committee Memberships, and Other Activities:
• List all, including years active
• List chronologically, beginning with earliest appointment
• If still active, list date as follows: 2011–

Professional and Society Memberships:
• List dates, offices held, and committee responsibilities
• List chronologically, beginning with earliest appointment

Invited Visiting Professorships:
• List dates, place, and professorship title
• List chronologically, beginning with earliest appointment

Presentations at National Meetings:
• List dates, meeting names, places, and topics
• List chronologically, beginning with earliest presentation

Presentations at International Meetings:
• List dates, meeting names, places, and topics
• List chronologically, beginning with earliest presentation

Intramural/In-house Presentations:
- Presentations at the physician's hospital or institutions; presentations, Mortality and Moribundity Conferences, or journal club meeting at Grand Rounds; or formal presentations to medical students
- List chronologically, beginning with earliest presentation

Research Grants:
- Grant number and title, time period
- List chronologically, beginning with earliest award

Hobbies/Interests/Civic Activities:
- List both medically and non-medically related activities

Publications – Journals:
- Published articles: List chronologically, beginning with earliest publication
- Use "In Press" for those articles accepted but not yet printed
- Use "Submitted" for those submitted but not yet accepted or rejected
- Use "In Preparation" for those written but not submitted

Publications – Abstracts, Editorials, Book Chapters:
- After the title, identify in parentheses whether the work is an abstract, an editorial, or a book chapter; put all abstracts in a separate grouping
- List chronologically, beginning with earliest publication

References (contact info for at least three):
- Colleagues; professors; mentors; former students

The following should NOT appear on your CV:
- Date of birth
- Sex/gender
- Family information
- Social Insurance, Social Security, or passport numbers
- Health Insurance number
- Education or awards prior to university unless relevant
- Details that you would not be willing to discuss in an interview

Source: Adapted from Alguire P, Whelan G, Rajput V, *The International Medical Graduate's Guide to US Medicine & Residency Training*, Philadelphia: ACP Press; 2009

BEFORE SIGNING ON: WHAT TO LOOK FOR IN RESIDENCY CONTRACTS[6]

The American Medical Association has published a document called "Guidelines for Housestaff Contracts or Agreements." Resident Doctors of Canada and the Committee of Interns and Residents (CIR) in the United States can also be contacted for contractual questions, although Canadian contracts tend to be pretty standard and uniform. Consult their general websites for links to this content.

Among the essential points to look for in a written agreement are the following:

- Specified salary year by year (which should be the same for all residents at your level)
- Work hours (including maximum call and days off)
- Available leave (including bereavement, illness, personal/family, educational – with duration specified)
- No limitations on off-duty involvements (i.e., you're free to moonlight)
- Holiday time details
- Contract termination procedures and appeal possibilities (related to quitting, transferring, or being fired)
- Transfer provisions (should your program close or amalgamate)
- Other benefits (living quarters, uniforms and laundry, meals, staff health services, pagers, lockers, library facilities)
- Policies related to sexual harassment, discrimination, disciplinary protocols, and grievances
- Flexibility regarding changing programs

REFERENCES

1 Gray K. Critical condition. *Details*, Sept. 2002: 149.
2 Carek PJ, Anderson KD. Residency selection process and the match: Does anybody believe anybody? *JAMA*. 2001;285(21):2784–5. http://dx.doi.org/10.1001/jama.285.21.2784-JMS0606-5-1. (This paper is still a classic.)
3 Raff MJ, Schwartz IS. An applicant's evaluation of a medical house officership. *N Engl J Med*. 1974;291(12):601–5. http://dx.doi.org/10.1056/NEJM197409192911204.
4 Van Dyke A, Seger AM. Finding, keeping, and revitalizing the meaning in family medicine. *Int J Psychiatry Med*. 2013;45(4):323–31. http://dx.doi.org/10.2190/PM.45.4.c.

5 *Strolling through the Match – The AAFP Students Guide to Residency Selection, 2015–2016*. American Academy of Family Physicians; 2011.
6 *Contracts: What You Need to Know*: http://www.ama-assn.org/ama/ama-wire/post/7-things-must-before-signing-employment-contract

CHAPTER THREE

Physician Heal Thyself: Taking Care of Your Body

THE VENDING MACHINE

Call nights as a medical student were always hectic. At first, it seemed like there was never a moment to sit down or even take a washroom break, and I went at least one whole night without one. But as I spent more time in the hospital at night, I came to recognize a rhythm that allowed for a quiet break around 3 AM every night.

There was a vending machine near one of the inpatient wards. I took to visiting at least once each call shift. I'd buy a bag of sour cream and onion chips and finish the whole thing on one of the nearby couches, half-listening to the reassuring snores and unsettling gasps of my patients down the hall. For a few minutes each night, I had a small sanctuary from the chaos.

When I became a senior resident, I started to bring all sorts of snacks to the room where my team reviewed our consults in an attempt to recreate that sanctuary, but this time bringing my interns and med students into it. What I brought reflected the stock of the hospital's drug store, which varied seasonally: iced tea in August; for some reason, popcorn in December. And always a couple big bags of chips!

Residents sometimes seem to forget, as they become used to ignoring physical cues including hunger, fatigue and bathroom breaks, that they themselves have bodies! This chapter offers some suggestions for keeping healthy physically during your years of training. Readers are also directed to a wonderful resource at the AMA – "A Physician's Guide to Personal Health Program"[1] (available at http://www.ama-assn.org), which guides you to make healthy lifestyle choices over time and reminds you to get regular check-ups/screening based on your age, health risk factors, and according to periodic medical exam guidelines.

SLEEP

TIP: *"I find it very beneficial to take a nap as soon as possible on call, e.g., if it's 5 PM and there are no pages, I can lie down until they come. This allows me to start refreshed, whenever."*

Historically, a lack of sleep has represented the most significant stress to physicians in training, who commonly worked 36-hour shifts as frequently as every second to every fourth day. While on duty, they averaged 2.7 hours of sleep. Although studies of shift workers abound,[2,3,4,5] relatively few have examined medical interns and residents. They have, however, shown a variety of effects of reduced sleep and fatigue, including the following: decreased mathematical ability, less accuracy in electrocardiogram reading, memory deficit, irritability, impaired concentration, depersonalization, inappropriate affect, and decreased cognitive performance and fine motor skills. One older study noted post-call car accidents in 35% of a sample of medical interns who were followed up for 1 month.[6] Since the last edition of this book, the

Table 3.1 More Resources on Sleep and Safety

• *Resident Duty Hours: Enhancing Sleep, Supervision and Safety.* National Academies Press, Washington, 2009
• Harvard Work Hours Health and Safety Group. At www.cirseiu.org

---

published evidence on how sleep deprivation leads to preventable errors (including needle-stick injuries) continues to grow.

Other professions have acknowledged categorically the risks attendant on sleep deprivation. Nurses, air pilots, air traffic and other transportation controllers and operators, army recruits, and nuclear inspectors and attendants all have regulated hours for reasons of individual and corporate safety. It is acknowledged by sleep experts that at least 5 hours of sleep are required for a worker to maintain cognitive and motor skills.[7] Medicine has been slow to acknowledge this risk to trainees and patients, in part because of the cost of replacement services and in part because of a traditional stoicism that equates forgoing sleep with dedication and opportunities for learning. However, in July 2003 the Accreditation Council for Graduate Medical Education (ACGME) implemented work-hours limitations, including a maximum of 80 hours work per week. Not surprisingly, some attending physicians have celebrated these changes. Others have pointed to their negative impact on learning and patient care, particularly in surgery.[8] (Note: New ACGME work hour rules actually went into effect in July 2011. The CIR has developed a Work Smart Tool Kit (http://www.cir.seiu.org/policy), which summarizes best practices from residency programs across the country.) Older studies had already demonstrated better cost and work efficiency when housestaff are less fatigued.[7] Newer research has confirmed that residents with modified working schedules are likely to make fewer medication errors, increase their productivity, and discharge patients faster. They also report enhanced career satisfaction and lower levels of exhaustion.[9,10]

Frequently changing or disrupted sleep schedules and sleep deprivation alter natural circadian rhythms and cause gastrointestinal complaints (e.g., indigestion, constipation, and dyspepsia), loss of appetite, mood swings, forgetfulness, chronic fatigue, and irritability. One study showed that up to 25% of all beeper pages were unimportant or unnecessary and actually interrupted patient care.[11] People with diabetes, epilepsy, depression, and respiratory disorders are at higher medical risk when they are deprived of sleep because of disrupted physiological cycles and altered efficacy or absorption of medications that are designed to coincide with these rhythms.

NODDING OFF

I couldn't believe it. I actually fell asleep in a patient's therapy session. I'd had a string of bad calls and just never seemed to catch up with my sleep. You probably know the feeling – your head is nodding, your eyes are closing, and no amount of tongue-biting, knee-pinching, shifting positions, or deep breathing is going to preserve wakefulness. The head bobs downward and that's that.

The patient was a man with schizophrenia, about 50.

I'll never forget my embarrassment or his kindness.

"Doc – you look exhausted. Make sure you take care of yourself."

Top 10 Cognitive and Neurobehavioral Effects of Fatigue[12,13,14]

1 Alertness and vigilance become unstable; lapses of attention increase.
2 Cognitive slowing occurs; time pressure increases errors.
3 Working memory declines.
4 Tasks may be begun well, but performance deteriorates with increasing rapidity.
5 Perseveration on ineffective solutions increases.
6 Neglect of activities judged to be nonessential (loss of situational awareness) grows.
7 Involuntary microsleep attacks occur.
8 Increased compensatory efforts required to remain effective.
9 Risks of critical errors and accidents increase.
10 Cognitive deficits can be masked by stimulation.

Although improved work hours have been in place in Canada for many years and have been adopted by programs in the United States, you can still enhance your sleep by applying a few strategies. Planning and conducting rounds before retiring, including giving clear instructions to nursing staff about pending laboratory results or vital-sign changes, can prevent unnecessary calls. If you are a senior resident and take call from home, go to bed early so you get some rest before the pages come in. Ideally, for in-house call, you should have your own room key and ready access to a telephone and bathroom with shower, and you should have the option to stay overnight in the room if late working hours make it inconvenient or unsafe for you to return home. In addition, it is not unreasonable to ask the head nurse or nursing supervisor to screen nursing requests before you are paged. Splitting the night with a colleague (midnight to 4 a.m., 4 a.m. to 8 a.m.) can ensure 4 hours of sleep without frequent interruption. Dedicated call-room facilities (i.e., not cloak-rooms) should be quiet, cleanly maintained, close to wards, and unshared (i.e., one person to a room). Ideally, support staff should be recruited to do the "scut" work, tasks that housestaff are usually expected to do at night. When possible, you should be paired with another resident to permit task splitting (e.g., emergency admission vs ward work), and you should be allowed to leave the next day after signing off patient care post-call, as specified in your contract. Insist on a proper handover.

TEN TIPS FOR FIRST AND SUBSEQUENT CALL NIGHTS

1 Pay close attention at evening sign-out rounds to particular problems with patients. Prioritize the sickest or most unstable patients. Make a "scut" list. Clarify management instructions from your senior resident.

2 Clarify with your senior how to proceed during call if you have questions and how to reach her to discuss cases. Clarify your role with the medical student as well. Do not hesitate to ask for teaching or help – that is why you are there.

3 Make sure your beeper works. Respond to pages quickly.

4 Prevent rather than treat. When you see a patient on a ward, ask if there are other concerns or problems while you're there. Make a list of results you need to check.

5 When you are called to assess someone, see the patient, and write a timed and dated note on every patient (as legal documentation and medical update). Leave clear instructions with

the nurse about when to call you again. If the nurse calls to inform you of something, discuss whether the patient needs to be seen.

6 Carry good pocket manuals or smartphone apps for differential diagnosis content and treatment guidelines. (See below.)

7 Organize your time strategically. Deal with all problems and review all laboratory and X-ray results service by service or floor by floor. Keep a detailed list. Assessing the patient and writing orders in the emergency department will save you travel time and even "scut" work, because most tests and blood sampling can be done there.

8 Although you have back-up and may not even be the first to see patients, discipline yourself to conduct thorough physical exams, differential diagnoses, work-ups, and treatment plans to avoid the temptation, especially when tired, to readily accept someone else's management. After residency you will not have this opportunity to test yourself under supervision.

9 Rehearse particular emergency management plans in your mind on the way to assess the patient. This will reduce anxiety and increase efficiency. *On-Call Principles and Protocols* is an excellent book that takes you step by step through key on-call problems and their management.[15]

10 There are also many useful apps that put info at your fingertips. Here's a sample list, by subject (some are free and some charge fees):

Subject	Smartphone Applications
Emergency Medicine	ACLS Advisor 2013 (free)
	WikEM Emergency Medicine (free)
	ERes – Emergency Medicine ($4.99)
Family Medicine	PalliCare.ca (free WebApp)
	AFP by Topic (free)
General	Medscape (free)
	Eye Chart Pro (free)
	Lab Values Pro ($2.99)
	MD on Call ($4.99)
	MedCalc Pro ($4.99)
	UpToDate (subscription)
	5-Minute Clinical Consult (subscription)

Subject	Smartphone Applications
Internal Medicine	ACC Pocket Guidelines (free)
	Harrison's Manual of Medicine (subscription)
Neurology	NeuroMind (free)
Obstetrics	Perfect OB wheel ($1.99)
Paediatrics	Paediatric Growth Chart (free)
	Pedi Safe ($0.99)
	Pedi STAT ($2.99)
Pharmacy	Epocrates (free)
	CPS Essentials ($39.99 annually)
	Lexi-comp (subscription)
Psychiatry	STAT Depression Score PHQ-9 (free)
	Psychiatry, Understanding Disease (free)

Consult your hospital or medical school librarian for additional (and sometimes discounted) apps, plus objective prescribing newsletters like the Medical Letter and the Cochrane Reviews.

11 Determine sign-over time the next morning and your role then (e.g., presentation of new admissions). Look after yourself the next day! Do not drive if you've been up over 16 hours! For tips on safe, effective hand-off techniques, go to www.ama-assn.org.

TIP: *"Many hospitals offer residents discounts on apps – ask what is available!"*

Tips for Regular Sleep[16]

You won't have control over how busy your shifts are, but there are some things you can do to protect your sleeping patterns:

- Sleep when you can. Follow your body's cues.
- Prioritize household tasks and check your e-mails later, *after* you get some sleep.
- Leave work at work. You've signed off and signed over care.
- Aim for a consistent post-call sleeping pattern or ritual.

- Take a 20-minute "wind down" period or warm bath before going to bed.
- Reduce the frequency of large meals and intake of greasy foods before retiring, but eat enough to prevent your waking hungry.
- Reduce or eliminate alcohol, caffeine, and tranquilizer consumption before retiring.
- Increase exercise, but not immediately before bedtime.
- Use the bed for sleep only; if you cannot sleep, do something else out of bed and delay your usual bedtime by 1 or 2 hours.
- Close the blinds.
- Shut off your smartphone/laptop. The light emitted by these devices disturbs sleep patterns/melatonin release!
- Use ear plugs, unplug the phone, and make sure the temperature and noise levels of your sleeping quarters are comfortable.
- Check out the LIFE Curriculum (www.lifecurriculum.info) for up-to-date articles and stats on managing sleep and fatigue:
  L – earning to address
  I – mpairment and
  F – atigue to
  E – nhance patient safety

TIP: "It should be made clear to on-call residents and nursing staff what tasks must be handled overnight and which can wait until morning. E.g., it should be made clear that most paperwork can wait until morning, etc. Night call should focus on patient care."

DIET

A recent study of residents and medical students showed that both groups failed to achieve recommended daily servings of fruits and vegetables. Stress and lack of sleep may suppress your appetite or lead to increased consumption of junk food or caffeine. Time pressure, and the poor quality or variety of hospital cafeteria food, often makes residents decide to skip meals entirely. The hypothalamic response to prolonged stress – such as occurs in residency – results in increased turnover of protein, carbohydrates, and fats and, if severe, may deplete vitamin and mineral reserves. This is itself a physiological stress factor. A lack of exposure to sunlight can lead to vitamin D deficiency.[17] Although nutrition guidelines now recommend a specific daily intake from each of the four food groups (dairy, meat and other protein, breads and cereals, and fruits and vegetables), several modifications can be useful.

Small frequent meals fit more easily than large ones into crowded schedules, produce less postprandial fatigue, and may lessen stress-induced dyspepsia or nausea, a common complaint of housestaff. Eating foods with a high fiber content will prevent changes in bowel habits, whereas a high level of fluid intake will prevent dehydration. Healthy snacks from the hospital cafeteria and vending machines should replace chocolate, pastries, and caffeinated beverages. Sweet snacks give only short-lived energy boosts, followed by rapid swings in blood sugar levels with a resultant "crash" or "let-down" fatigue. Caffeine may be tempting if you are tired, but it may produce increased anxiety, tremors, and irritability!

Many healthy foods can be requested of the hospital and stocked in the interns' lounge or lockers so they are available when meals are missed (see below). Vitamin supplementation remains a controversial issue because there is no definitive proof that increased emotional stress depletes nutritional stores. A "B-C-E-D vitamin/mineral" complex may, however, be useful in the face of irregular eating habits and skipped meals. Certainly a woman with a tendency toward anemia will have impaired energy levels if she does not receive an iron supplement.

Fuel-Efficient Snacks

If you have to eat on the run, here are some fuel-efficient snacks:

- Fruit (apples and pears)
- Low-fat yogurt, cottage cheese, skim milk (high in protein, may boost energy)
- Whole wheat bagels, bread, and toast (with peanut butter)
- Dried fruit (e.g., raisins)
- Graham crackers and whole-wheat ginger snaps
- Carrots and celery
- Pretzels
- Nuts
- Cheese slices
- Protein shakes

Eating Strategies

Keep track of your weight and nutritional status on a regular basis. Here are some helpful eating strategies:

- Make sure you hydrate properly (6–8 glasses of water/day).
- Eat small meals frequently, and don't skip meals.
- Have only light meals before sleep.
- Eat a diet composed of 55% carbohydrates, less than 30% fat, and 15% protein.
- Consider vitamin supplementation.
- Decrease your intake of caffeine, tobacco, alcohol, fatty foods, and simple carbohydrates.
- Increase your intake of complex carbohydrates.
- Avoid fad dieting.
- Pack healthy, high-protein snacks for on-call periods.

BAD HABITS

Increased levels of stress, as described in chapter 1, can provoke increased alcohol consumption and use of cigarettes and of both illicit and prescription drugs. Cigarette smoking may suppress your appetite and results in increased vitamin C requirements. Alcohol binges during time off may produce a hangover with characteristic symptoms of headache, nausea, and decreased reaction time, but they also may result in dehydration and vitamin B depletion. The street drugs most often used by housestaff are stimulants (cocaine and amphetamines) and appetite suppressants, but prescription narcotics (like oxycodone) and tranquilizers (especially benzodiazepines and sleeping pills) are used as well. Residents are also abusing modafinil (Alertec/Provigil) to stay awake. Drug use and abuse, and resources for finding help, are discussed in chapter 6 (see "The Impaired Colleague").

OTHER STRESS BUSTERS

Tips for time management[18]

1 Read emails/touch paperwork only once. This will help you declutter and prevent you from postponing tasks or losing information.

2 Make task lists every day. Indicate their priority – i.e., what's urgent, what can wait, what imminent deadlines exist.

3 Keep your paper/virtual calendar up to date regarding social and professional engagements. Use the "month at a glance" feature to scope an overview and to review deadlines and other important dates.

4 Develop useful routines: make a point of completing notes after every patient visit, dictating summaries the day of discharge, picking a regular time to review lab results and check your mail.

5 Don't be idle! If you have a waiting period or a patient no-show, check your to-do list and get something done. Don't fiddle with your phone!

6 Maximize rounding efficiency:
   - Start and end on time.
   - Set goals.
   - Review/track down lab results prior to rounds.
   - Be ready to introduce your patient and present your case succinctly and respectfully.

For more tips, read "The time management guide – a practical handbook for physicians by physicians," available online at www.royal college.ca.

EXERCISE

Regular exercise seems almost impossible to schedule for most interns and residents because of fatigue and time pressure. It takes some inventiveness to incorporate exercise into a busy routine. Aerobic exercise, for periods of 20 to 30 minutes, three times a week, is an ideal solution to emotional stress because it enhances relaxation through endorphin release, decreases depressive symptoms, increases energy levels, improves sleep, dampens the fight-or-flight response, and improves the physiological response to emotional and physical challenge. Many residents walk, ride, or run to work and climb stairs at work rather than take the elevator. Others buy an exercycle or rowing machine for home use, live in an apartment complex with a pool or sports facilities, or join a gym near the hospital. Others arrange to use facilities in the hospital such as the pool or Nautilus machines in the physiotherapy department.

Besides regular exercise, various simple techniques of relaxation can significantly reduce physical tension, anxiety, and fatigue.[19] You may also want to learn more about yoga, meditation, and mindfulness stress reduction. Some hospitals even offer free classes for staff. One study showed that offering access to a no-fee hospital-based fitness center to surgical residents improved their productivity and quality of work.[17]

SIMPLE RELAXATION EXERCISES

Abdominal Breathing

Most people under stress take frequent, quick, shallow breaths using only their diaphragms. To change this pattern, use the abdomen and take deeper breaths, by letting your belly fall out. Breaking inspiration into sniffs to the count of four and then exhaling to the count of four soon induces relaxation. Each breathing cycle takes eight seconds; the appearance of sighing signals that the exercise is working.

Shoulder Shrugs

Shrugging your shoulders reduces tension in the upper body, which is usually affected during periods of stress. Inhale while pulling your shoulders up toward your head; rotate your shoulders so that your shoulder blades come together and exhale while letting your shoulders fall back down. Three to five repetitions in a sitting or standing position usually result in quick relief.

Head Rolls

Relieve neck tension by exhaling while letting your chin fall toward your chest. Breathe in while rotating your head to the right and to the back, and then exhale while rotating your head to the left and forward to your chest. Repeat three to five cycles in a sitting or standing position.

Progressive Muscular Relaxation

This is a useful technique that can also be taught to patients who feel under stress. Alternately tense and relax each muscle group in sequence from your toes up to your buttocks; extend or puff out your abdomen and chest; finally, progressively tense and relax your fingers, arms, shoulders, and facial muscles. Do this exercise while you are lying down in a quiet place, inhaling during the muscular tension phase of a few seconds and exhaling during a few seconds of letting the muscles go limp. Five minutes should be sufficient for this total-body relaxation exercise.

REMAINING MINDFUL[20]

Mindfulness involves bringing one's complete attention to the present experience, on a moment-to-moment basis. This allows you to observe mental and bodily experiences more clearly and without judgment, and to put them in perspective.

- Check your breathing throughout the day. Take 10 full, deep breaths.
- Watch your posture whenever you move from standing to sitting, lying down or walking. What is your body telling you?
- Check in with your five senses – what are you seeing, hearing, tasting, touching, smelling?
- Listen to others without interruption or judgment. When it's your turn, make your point calmly, with your body relaxed.
- Check your muscle tone during the day. Are your muscles stiff, sore, tight, relaxed? Stretch out the tension.
- Whenever possible, eat slowly. Taste. Chew. Pay attention!
- Make a point of paying attention to daily, even routine, activities (instead of doing them on automatic pilot). Observe yourself brushing your teeth, washing the dishes, tying your shoelaces. Be present. Be here, now!
- Observe your thoughts and feelings in a given moment – whether irritated, amused, overwhelmed, happy. Name the feeling for yourself. Take a breath and don't judge what you're feeling. At the same time, don't act on it or speak out without reflecting.

PROTECTING YOUR PHYSICAL HEALTH

- Get a family doctor! Your program might be able to help you find one.
- Update your immunizations. Arrange for a diphtheria and tetanus booster if your last vaccination was more than 10 years ago.

- Consult your Postgraduate Medical Education (PGME) office to determine which vaccinations are obligatory. As an example, arrange for tuberculin skin testing, so that you know your status and can be assessed after exposure, and followed up on or treated if necessary. Inquire about hospital policy on TB enforcement. (The US Centers for Disease Control suggest yearly TB testing for healthcare workers.)
- Arrange for measles, polio, and rubella vaccination if you have not been vaccinated or if you have no history of any of these diseases.
- Update tetanus/ diphtheria boosters.
- Women of child-bearing age should have a rubella hemagglutination inhibition test to determine their immune status.
- Mumps and varicella (chicken pox) vaccinations are optional, but are strongly advised in the absence of previous vaccination or documented disease. Influenza vaccination is often mandatory, but is strongly advised for those at increased risk of, for example, asthma, diabetes, severe anemia, immunodeficiency, and heart or renal disease. Consider getting the acellular pertussis vaccine as well. Discuss these vaccinations with your staff health office.
- Hepatitis B vaccine is strongly advised and should be provided free of charge by your hospital. Both plasma-derived and recombinant forms have been proved safe and effective. Your work as a resident puts you at risk of contracting hepatitis B; do not take the chance.
- Hepatitis A vaccine is also available and recommended.
- Prevent lower-back injuries by avoiding excessive leaning over a patient; raise the bed, not the patient. Pay attention to posture when you are sitting or standing for prolonged periods. Obtain help when lifting patients or equipment. Get close to the patient or object and lift with your legs. Ask an orderly to show you how.
- Avoid radiation exposure by standing at least 18 meters from portable X-ray equipment. Ask for a portable radiation meter if you are working in an area of high exposure (e.g., radiology).
- Request adequate training for the handling of toxic substances (e.g., anti-neoplastic agents) and information on local "right to know" laws about exposure to toxic materials.
- Arrange for a mask fitting in preparation for exposure to airborne infections.

- Review your institution's pandemic/ disaster protocols. (Sample guidelines can be found at http://residentdoctors.ca.)
- Do not drive a car or ride your bicycle if drowsy!

PROTECTING YOURSELF FROM PHYSICAL VIOLENCE[21,22]

Trainees often forget that distressed patients may lose control and lash out physically. You can learn to recognize these signs of imminent danger:

By Patient History

- Past history of violence or criminal involvement
- Threats of violence
- Poor social functioning (e.g., conflict with authority, job/school conflicts)
- History of childhood sexual or physical abuse
- Personality disorders (antisocial or borderline)

By Diagnosis

- Alcohol or drug intoxication or withdrawal
- Acute mania or psychosis (including command hallucinations)
- Organic brain syndrome or delirium
- Seizures (temporal lobe, partial or complex)

Behavioral

- Loud, threatening speech
- Tense, clenched posture
- Agitation or restlessness
- Pacing, easy to startle
- Rapid breathing
- Violent gestures (pounding the table, pointing)

STRATEGIES TO ENSURE SAFETY

- Find out about your hospital's safety policy and determine what rights you have as an employee.

- Familiarize yourself with security measures already in place (video cameras, alarm buzzers; weapon and firearm checks by security; hospital emergency "code" protocols).
- Review hospital procedures for physical restraint.
- Warn others of high-risk behaviors if you witness them. Don't allow a situation to escalate.
- Watch how you dress. Accessories, ties, pens, pins, necklaces, chains, and scissors are all potential weapons. Long hair can be pulled.
- Be courteous and non-provocative regardless of the patient's behavior. Do not lecture, condescend, or express annoyance.
- Make sure the examining area is well lit and clutter-free (e.g., with no throwable objects).
- Never stand between the patient and the door, and when sitting make sure *you* have the closest access to the exit or door.
- If you feel you are in danger, do not continue the exam or interview. Leave at once and caution security.
- When in doubt about a patient, call a support staff member or request the presence of a third party.
- Do not stare at, point at, or touch an angry patient.
- If a patient is agitated, request physical restraint during your examination, especially if drawing blood. Avoid needle-stick injuries!
- Make sure your call room door is locked.
- Be cautious when leaving hospital grounds at night. If in doubt, take a taxi or request that a security guard accompany you to your car.
- Suggestions for handling disruptive colleagues can be found in chapter 6.

Avoiding Viral and Bacterial Infections

- Follow stringently all isolation and hand-washing precautions for both your safety and that of your patients. Keep your hands away from your eyes and face to reduce the incidence of viral infections. Use antibacterial hand gel throughout the day.

- Reduce your risk of needle-stick injuries by *never* recapping needles; never manipulate used scalpel blades without an instrument; never leave used needles around (e.g., on beds); dispose of all sharp objects in an appropriate container that is not full; and seek help for blood-related procedures when a patient is agitated. Should you sustain a needle-stick injury, let the wound bleed, wash it with soap and water, disinfect it with alcohol, and then immediately call the staff health unit for follow-up procedures. Protocols for post-HIV exposure (i.e., drug therapy) now exist and you should request treatment if indicated.
- Make sure that all equipment you use is adequately maintained, disinfected, and sterilized.
- Use precautions against human immunodeficiency virus infection.[23] Follow the universal blood and body-fluid precautions and recommendations concerning handling of body fluids and procedures for using gloves and washing hands listed below.

Universal Blood and Body-Fluid Precautions

Body fluids for which gloves followed by hand-washing are recommended (visit www.cdc.gov for updates):

- Blood
- Blood-contaminated fluids
- Sperm
- Cerebrospinal fluid
- Pleural fluid
- Pericardial fluid
- Peritoneal fluid
- Synovial fluid
- Amniotic fluid

Body fluids for which gloves are not recommended (if not contaminated by blood), but hand-washing *is* recommended:

- Saliva
- Stools, diarrhea

- Vomitus
- Tears
- Nasal secretions
- Oral secretions

Procedures for which gloves followed by hand-washing are recommended:

- Intubation
- Bronchoscopy
- Dental procedures
- Wound irrigation
- Phlebotomy
- Finger and/or heel stick
- Vascular catheter placement
- Tracheotomy suctioning
- Rinsing of used instruments
- Lumbar puncture
- Amniocentesis
- Puncture of other cavities

Masks and eye barrier protection should be used *whenever* splattering is likely. Diaper changing is usually done without gloves but followed immediately by hand washing.

Illness during Training

Residents and interns are not immune from health problems, although they like to believe that they are. The following suggestions are made to residents who become ill during training.

- Do not come to work if you have an acute, infectious illness. "Presenteeism" is a risk to your fellow residents.
- Do not use denial to avoid receiving the medical attention you need.
- Maintain a good link with your treating physician, who can see or refer you, or admit you to hospital quickly.

- Do not self-treat and do not play "doctor games" with your physician about knowledge and control issues. Find someone competent and caring and let yourself be cared for; relinquish the need for total control.
- Do not expect special treatment or automatic professional courtesy. An inflated sense of entitlement may complicate your relationship with your caregivers.
- Take the time you need to get better. Let your physician manage any administrative pressures from your superiors that may hinder your recovery. Most contracts allow for sick leave, so you will not be penalized for absence from work.
- Never self-prescribe medications or order investigations – see the classic article by GE Vaillant: Physician cherish thyself: The hazards of self-prescribing.[24]
- If you are HIV-positive yourself, read "The legal rights and obligations of HIV-infected health care workers" by the Gay and Lesbian Medical Association (www.glma.org) or contact your provincial or state medical association for current policies.

WHY DO WE WAIT SO LONG TO OBTAIN HELP?

It's both paradoxical and ironic that physicians who advocate healthy lifestyles to their patients often neglect their own health, and ignore early warning signs of significant physical or mental illness. Doctors are forced to embrace a level of stoicism and perfectionism in their training and often come to ignore their own physical cues. They may believe that their white coat somehow magically protects from them from serious illness and use denial around symptoms they would investigate and treat actively in a patient.

Doctors are often pressed for time, may have significant educational debts, and are afraid of taking time off work or being placed (or forced) onto disability leave. Many residents and fellows do not have their own family doctor, and this can delay obtaining appropriate care and specialty referrals.

TIP: *"I know now that if anyone in medicine asks me for help that I should act right away. Chances are they've been sitting on it for some time."*

When it comes to issues of burn-out or mental illness, doctors are understandably reluctant to be treated by colleagues they know within their hospital network as they fear confidentiality may be breached and they may be stigmatized. Their families may have made sacrifices to educate them or to permit the building of a practice and the physician may fear losing status and idealization from family members.

Furthermore, many physicians fear that their health concerns will be reported to licensing bodies, thus damaging their careers and earning potential. Promoting the role of physician health programs (PHPs) and residency well-being programs is a good way to reduce stigma and to encourage good self-care. Information on local PHPs can be found in chapter 13.

REFERENCES

1 At http://www.ama-assn.org/ama/pub/physician-resources/public-health/promoting-healthy-lifestyles/healthier-life-steps-program/physicians-personal-health.page.

2 Colford JM, McPhee SJ. The raveled sleeve of care. *JAMA*. 1989;261:889–93. http://dx.doi.org/10.1001/jama.1989.03420060105041.

3 Leighton K, Livingston M. Fatigue in doctors. *Lancet*. 1983;321(8336):1280. http://dx.doi.org/10.1016/S0140-6736(83)92732-0.

4 Friedman RC, Bigger JT, Kornfeld DS. The intern and sleep loss. *N Engl J Med*. 1971;285(4):201–3. http://dx.doi.org/10.1056/NEJM197107222850405.

5 Friedman RC, Bigger JT, Kornfeld DS. Psychological problems associated with sleep deprivation in interns. *J Med Educ*. 1973;48:436–41.

6 Katz S. Shifting gears: Shift work's assault on our biological rhythms. *Medical Post*, 3 Oct. 1989; 11–12, 48. These findings were replicated in a CIR survey reported in March 2001.

7 Swift D. Humane schedules for residents, interns helps reduce risk of errors. *Medical Post*. 1989;26:47.

8 Ahmed N, Devitt KS, Keshet I, et al. A systematic review of the effects of resident duty hour restrictions in surgery: Impact on resident wellness, training, and patient outcomes. *Ann Surg*. 2014;259(6):1041–53. http://dx.doi.org/10.1097/SLA.0000000000000595.

9 Veasey S, Rosen R, Barzansky B, et al. Sleep loss and fatigue in residency training: A reappraisal. *JAMA*. 2002;288(9):1116–24. http://dx.doi.org/10.1001/jama.288.9.1116.

10 Goitein L, Shanafelt TD, Wipf JE, et al. The effects of work-hour limitations on resident well-being, patient care, and education in an internal

medicine residency program. *Arch Intern Med.* 2005;165(22):2601–6. http://dx.doi.org/10.1001/archinte.165.22.2601.

11 Blum NJ, Lieu TA. Interrupted Care. *Am J Dis Child.* 1992;146:806–8. http://dx.doi.org/10.1001/archpedi.1992.02160190038016.

12 Dinges D. Cited in *CIR News*, Dec. 2001.

13 Hochberg MS, Berman RS, Kalet AL, et al. The stress of residency: Recognizing the signs of depression and suicide in you and your fellow residents. *Am J Surg.* 2013;205(2):141–6. http://dx.doi.org/10.1016/j.amjsurg.2012.08.003.

14 Knight JM. Physiological and neurobiological aspects of stress and their relevance for residency training. *Acad Psychiatry.* 2013;37(1):6–10. http://dx.doi.org/10.1176/appi.ap.11100187.

15 Marshall SA, Ruedy J. *On-Call Principles and Protocols.* 4th ed. Philadelphia: Saunders; 2004.

16 Watson DT, Long WJ, Yen D, et al. Health promotion program: A resident well-being study. *Iowa Orthop.* 2009;29:83–7.

17 Haney EM, Stadler D, Bliziotes MM. Vitamin D insufficiency in internal medicine residents. *Calcif Tissue Int.* 2005;76(1):11–6. http://dx.doi.org/10.1007/s00223-004-0025-0.

18 Bong-You R. *The Residency Survival Manual.* Yarmouth, MA: Morgan Bay Productions; 2004.

19 Borysenko J. *Minding the Body, Mending the Mind.* New York: Bantam; 1988.

20 Place S, Talen M. Creating a culture of wellness: Conversations, curriculum, concrete resources, and control. *Int J Psychiatry Med.* 2013;45(4):333–44. http://dx.doi.org/10.2190/PM.45.4.d.

21 Durso C, George SC. Guns 'n' doctors. *New Physician*, Dec. 1994. At www.amsa.org/tnp

22 Liss G, McCaskell L. Violence in the workplace. *Can Med Assoc J.* 1994;151:1243–6.

23 See www.cdc.gov for updates.

24 Vaillant GE. Physician cherish thyself: The hazards of self-prescribing. *JAMA.* 1992;267(17):2373–83. http://dx.doi.org/10.1001/jama.1992.03480170099038.

Staying Whole: Maximizing Supports and Finding Balance

Chapter 3 suggested ways of safeguarding physical health by improving your eating, sleeping, exercise habits, resilience, and stress-busting. This chapter discusses two important strategies for protecting your mental health: establishing adequate support systems and maximizing a sense of personal control and balance.

Relationships with family and friends are discussed in chapter 5, since most residents tend to go to these individuals when experiencing difficulty during training. Other types of support that you might not have considered are available from the following people, groups, and organizations.

MAXIMIZING SUPPORT AT WORK

Family Physician

Surprisingly, many residents and physicians do not have their own physicians, preferring to treat themselves or somehow expecting preferential care from colleagues, often with problematic results. (As mentioned in the previous chapter, this may in fact result from our own fears about being a patient.) One study of internal-medicine residents in a US school revealed that 37% had no primary care physician and 12% acted as their own doctor![1] Plan early. Before beginning your training, find a family physician who will treat you as a patient but can adapt to your erratic schedule. He or she can be an invaluable referral source for quick initial assessment and treatment, sick notes, stress management, and support. Your program may keep a list of local doctors willing to see residents.

Chief Resident

The chief resident should be your advocate, open to feedback about your rotations, and a mediator between residents and staff. He or she can initiate you into the conditions and customs in a new hospital or ward setting, arrange coverage when you are absent, ease necessary contacts with superiors, and field your call requests for the night duty roster.

TIP: "The chain of command and people who can provide backup should always be clear. E.g., a junior resident should know what senior residents and members of other services (i.e., ICU, anesthesia) are available to help as needed, how to contact staff, etc."

Senior Resident or Fellow

Local politics aside, this person can be a source of teaching, support, conflict resolution, and service orientation, and can help you organize your work. Do not hesitate to ask this person questions.

Residency Program Directors and the Postgraduate Medical Education (PGME) Office

Many residents unfortunately do not get to know their residency program director at either the hospital or the university program level. This important ally can provide information about rotations, electives, evaluations, exams, training options, and requirements. She can handle grievances about rotation abuses, requests for absences, or program changes, and can make recommendations about staff conflicts or learning difficulties. Schedule at least two appointments a year with the program director for feedback and to discuss your progress and career plans. As well, the PGME office can provide resources and usually has an orientation guide with key information on politics and procedures, including codes of conduct, intimidation and harassment protocols, and details on the accommodation of special physical or learning needs. Some schools even have a resident advocacy committee to help address concerns.[2]

The Postgraduate Medical Education Office

The postgraduate medical education office can provide information on training requirements and program resources and may also be able to link you with a residency advocate or ombudsman.

Hospital Housestaff Association or Resident Representative

This person should address such issues as duties, call frequency, adequacy of supervision, staff relations, leaves of absence, benefits, legal protection, and potential political action. All Canadian teaching institutions have a representative of the provincial hospital housestaff association in addition to a residency program delegate. Fewer than 25% of US programs are formally unionized, but your hospital may have residency representatives to the hospital or program administration (see chapter 13 for further union resources).

Religious Representatives

Scheduling a visit or having lunch with the hospital chaplain, priest, imam, rabbi, or other religious representative can help you to explore existential questions and clarify dilemmas that arise during the dark nights of the soul that many residents experience. Visits from them can also help some patients; ask your patients if they would like a visit arranged.

Hospital Ethics Consultant

Residents may feel ill at ease following certain recommendations of a senior person or experience moral conflicts in treating patients. These circumstances create great stress. Most teaching hospitals and universities have an ethics consultant who can be asked about such cases and invited to give formal or informal seminars.

Hospital Lawyer or Risk Manager

This person can answer questions about consent, confidentiality, incompetence, and termination of treatment, either personally or in requested lectures. Contact with this person is especially important in the United States, where the high risk of malpractice suits lends cogency to arguments for reducing residents' hours and improving working conditions.

Hospital Employee Assistance Programs, Provincial/ State Medical Association Hotline, or Local Physician Well-being Committee

The people from these services can tell you in confidence how to find help for yourself or your colleagues should someone increasingly resort to drugs or alcohol or to other maladaptive behavior in response to stress. One excellent example is Ontario's PAIRO Helpline at 1-866-HelpDoc (435-7362). These individuals can also refer you, when necessary, to the state or provincial physician health program (PHP) and to occupational health, career counseling, professional coaching, and/or human resources in your hospital. (See resource lists in chapter 13.) The mandate and breadth of offering of PHPs continues to expand with an emphasis on wellness, career enhancement and satisfaction, and building resilience rather than managing impairment.

Other Hospital Professionals

A hospital is a complex organization of professionals and nonprofessionals working together daily. You can have satisfying, friendly exchanges with any of them. If you can avoid taking a "physician-in-charge" stance, it is possible to develop relations of collaboration, camaraderie, and even friendship with paging operators, security guards, kitchen and cleaning staff, secretaries, orderlies, and X-ray and laboratory technologists, as well as with nurses, pharmacists, social workers, dietitians, and occupational and physical therapists. Take the time to learn their names and build a sense of community.

Mentor

Young professionals in any discipline need at least one mentor (a superior who is guide, tutor, and even friend) to help form their identity. Although some residency programs assign tutors, you may wish or be obliged to find a mentor yourself. In the latter case, ask an inspiring lecturer or attending physician for a meeting or request from the residency program director a list of people with similar clinical and research interests. Mentors are usually but not necessarily older people and may be of the same sex as you. This last characteristic may be an important factor in the process of identification that takes place in such a relationship. Many residents prefer same-sex mentors.

Finding a mentor or career coach may be the single most important step you take in obtaining professional support during residency. He or she can encourage you when you feel overwhelmed by your duties, buffer disillusionment, and help you with your career decisions.

A GOOD MENTOR

A good mentor is someone who:

- Is experienced, enthusiastic, sparks your interest, and can skillfully guide your reading and learning.
- Provides a role model with respect to manner, professional identity, ethics concerns, and lifestyle, and sees medicine as a vocation, not just a job.
- Maintains clear boundaries and directs you for added support and consultation where needed.
- Is patient, nonjudgmental, and non-evaluative (is not grading you for your work).
- Has artistic, research, and/or clinical interests similar to yours.
- Is flexible with time, does not compete with you, and is not threatened by your enthusiasm or intelligence.
- Is well connected to resource networks and key workers in your field.
- Will help you choose a subspecialty or fellowship and develop leadership skills.

Remember that we all need/can provide mentorship over the span of a medical career, so nurture those relationships over time!

Psychotherapists and Counselors

Many residents, particularly those in psychiatry programs, begin a psychotherapeutic exploration during residency, often as a result of crisis (career uncertainty, substance abuse, depression, or decreasing performance) and sometimes because they believe such work will make them happier people and better physicians. Your family physician, residency program director, hospital or provincial or state physician well-being committee, physician hotline, or you yourself, privately, can usually arrange a referral. Some residency programs include funded counseling networks or access to employee assistance programs (EAPs). Don't let fear or stigma stand in the way of getting help.

Select a therapist carefully; as one of my colleagues in Montreal observed, "You don't get to pick your parents, so you'd better be careful finding a therapist." Interview prospective therapists about philosophy and length of treatment, an active versus a silent approach, availability of a professional rate, and flexibility of hours, all the while assessing personal fit or compatibility ("Is this someone I can talk to?"). Decide whether you want support or a perceptive examination of conflicts, and whether you want to do short-term work or to keep the therapy open-ended. Make a contract with the therapist that sets goals, expectations, and basic ground rules (rates, attendance, holidays, cancellations, etc.).

The logistics of attending therapy sessions during residency are complex but not impossible to manage. If your residency program director has provided the referral, he or she may help you to be seen quickly and can be quoted during rotations as supporting therapy work. The referral source and therapist will keep your work confidential, but you will still have to explain absences to your senior or chief resident. Explain only as much as you want to, but at the least indicate that your work should not suffer from regular 1- to 2-hour absences each week. Having a therapist in the same hospital or nearby is an obvious advantage. Remember to keep any receipts for income tax purposes and to discuss with your therapist whether treatment will restrict medical and/or disability insurance access later on.

SUPPORT GROUPS[3-11]

Resident Support Groups

Some very worthwhile friendships form during internship and residency because of the intensity of the shared experience, the similar goals, and the countless hours that residents spend together. Many residents unfortunately miss the opportunity of giving and receiving informal peer support because they are competitive or believe they have to appear all-knowing and omnipotent. They are reluctant to discuss anxiety, sickness, self-doubt, or feelings of failure and loss after a patient's death. Build a community, and not just with residents in your own residency program. Link up with colleagues from other clinical disciplines. Allow yourself to let off steam, because it will help open exchange and normalize the many feelings that get stirred up in all residents during training. Ask for help when you need it, cover for each other, do favors, talk through intense shared experiences together (like the death of a patient). Build in play time (like a movie night or a softball game). All these activities are rewarding and protective. When you are a senior, look out for those under you, recognize their anxiety, and ask them to talk about such key experiences as the first night of call. Be a role model by showing that residents should talk about such things. Always set up an orientation or "boot camp" for new interns or new residents on your service.

TIP: *"I would advise performing the most cognitively intensive tasks earlier in the night (e.g., interpreting a blood gas, reassessing a patient) if at all possible, and performing less intense ones (checking bloodwork where critical values are highlighted, co-signing orders) later."*

The literature on resident stress and impairment has established the usefulness of a variety of formal group experience for residents, including exercise programs.[4,5] Women's groups, spouses' groups, couples' groups, trainee-staff retreats, first-year orientation weeks or months, medical society memberships, process or Balint-type groups, and peer/process support groups have all been used with success in teaching centers across North America. They may be optional or an established part of the program, time-limited or open, led by a behavioral scientist or self-run, and held weekly, monthly, or semiannually. Interns in particular benefit from such groups because they help to manage the stress of the first postgraduate year.

Recent innovations in resident support include boot camps with content on handling emergencies and particularly stressful situations,[6] transition to residency workshops and simulations for graduating med students,[7,8] communication and stress management training,[9] "Neighborhood Watch" initiatives, and formalized lectures on issues like personal development, coping with stress and maintaining balance.[10]

Nowadays, residents also keep in touch by blogging, texting, and contributing to trainee websites (both intranet and Internet), forming virtual support communities.[11]

Resident Support Structure – What's Ideal?

The Accreditation Council for Graduate Medical Education (ACGME) now requires that support services be available to all residents. Robert Levey in his literature review in *Academic Medicine*[12] highlights the stressors cited previously in chapter 1, but also mentions the dilemmas faced by international medical graduates (IMGs), residents who are matched to programs they don't want, pregnant and minority residents, and those with learning difficulties. Levey describes the following ingredients of an ideal assistance service:

- Confidentiality
- Support from program staff
- Short-term counseling or stress management for trainees and their family members
- An objective third-party referral service
- Ongoing follow-up for severely stressed residents
- Social activities and retreats
- Support groups for residents and family members
- Stress management seminars
- Child care and financial resources

The various residency program syllabuses and information networks now list and describe the support programs available at every hospital or university setting. See chapter 2 for information on choosing a healthy residency program. All of this information should figure highly in the choice of a program. My hope is that Canadian and US residents will share successful strategies about what works so that programs don't have to reinvent the wheel each time.

Housestaff Representation

Political support and influence are necessary to change the many stressful conditions now prevalent in the residency experience. All Canadian residents are employed by provincial agencies and represented by provincial housestaff associations, which provide uniform contracts. The Canadian Association of Internes and Residents (now http://residentdoctors.ca) has been serving as the umbrella organization for all provincial housestaff associations, excluding the Fédération des Médecins Résidents du Québec (FMRQ), since 1970. Residency groups from across the world have consulted CAIR because of its pioneering approaches to protecting the well-being of residents. In 2015, CAIR changed its name to Resident Doctors of Canada (RDoC).

The RDoC executive committee consists of provincially elected members who meet three times a year in different Canadian cities and sit on several of the major medical bodies, including the Canadian Medical Association (CMA), the Canadian Medical Protective Association (CMPA), the Royal College of Physicians and Surgeons of Canada (RCPSC), the College of Family Physicians of Canada, and various government and accreditation committees (e.g., on national manpower). RDoC publishes the *Canadian Housestaff* newsletter and other communications, which residents can request, and has a useful library on its website. It has also been active in sharing its expertise with its US counterparts, as they have been at the forefront with respect to addressing residents' rights and working conditions.

The situation in the United States historically has been quite different. Residents are generally hired and paid by their specific hospital center, and only 25% of hospitals have official housestaff unions with collective agreements. The Committee of Interns and Residents (CIR – www.cirseiu.org) is the oldest and largest housestaff union in the United States, with chapters across the country, and has an affiliation with the Service Employees' International Union (SEIU), which is the single largest American union of health employees. The CIR's services include consultation and advice on contract negotiations, union formation, and policies regarding call duties, licensing, funding, debt repayment, and other housestaff issues (e.g., quality of training and quality of life for patients and residents). The CIR publishes a newspaper, *CIR Vitals* (www.cirvitals.org), which monitors these concerns and carries information packets on affirmative action, IMG rights, legislative issues, public sector healthcare, contract negotiation, parenting issues, setting up a housestaff organization, limiting hours, improving safety and quality control, and issues like residency and AIDS.

Historically, other examples of more local unions could be found at the University of Michigan and the University of Colorado, as well as specific county hospitals (like Cook County Hospital in Chicago). Other schools and hospitals have housestaff associations that organize collectively on behalf of residents, but don't bargain and are not recognized under the National Labor Relations Act, as unions are. (The term "union" can be a dirty word for many medical educators because they feel any call for strikes or labor action would be "unethical" and not "physician-like.")

A few medical residents in the United States may still not be protected in any systematic way from local abuses in working conditions, especially in some of the southern states. Some residents have no board representation at the administrative level in the hospitals where they work. Challenges to contract violation must be fought individually. As well, many states and hospital corporations choose to see residents as students rather than as employees, thereby blocking the possibility for union formation and recognition. Nonetheless, many residents and academic staff are ambivalent about what "unionization" actually means within a profession like medicine and what impact it has on the doctor–patient relationship.

The American Medical Association plays a significant role in the lives of residents in the United States. Its Resident and Fellow Section (RFS), with over 35,000 members, is the largest organization of medical residents in the United States and contributes directly to the AMA policy-making process. Its journal (*JAMA*) publishes a regular column called "On Call" (email: oncall@ama-assn.org) that highlights key developments affecting young physicians in terms of legislation, debt repayment, practice formation, and training. The AMA also offers expert speakers to help residents explore their representational options (for information consult the AMA website, www.ama-assn.org).

Other organizations of interest to interns and residents in the United States include the following:

- American Medical Student Association (AMSA – www.amsa.org), which describes itself as "the largest and oldest independent association representing physicians-in-training, including pre-medical students, medical students, interns and residents. Founded in 1950 to provide an opportunity for medical students to participate in organized medicine, AMSA began as the Student American Medical Association under the auspices of the American Medical Association (AMA). In 1967, AMSA formally ended its affiliation with the AMA and has since remained an independent organization. Governed by a student Board of Trustees, much of the association's energy today is focused on reforming the medical education system, improving work conditions and developing physician leadership for the 21st century. AMSA has nearly 30,000 members in 168 chapters." AMSA also publishes the *New Physician*, a magazine on training issues and members work with CIR. (There is now a joint CIR-AMSA one-year fellowship.)[13]

- The Accreditation Council for Graduate Medical Education (ACGME – www.acgme.org) is the only accrediting body for the more than 6,000 residency training programs in the United States. Representatives from the AMA, the American Board of Medical Specialties, the American Hospital Association, and the Association of American Medical Colleges (AAMC), along with resident representatives and representatives from the public sector and the federal government, make up this body. The ACGME insists that every residency program have a grievance policy overseen by the hospital graduate medical education committee. It also investigates complaints about programs. They have wonderful web resources on multiple topics for residents.
- The AAMC (www.aamc.org) has an Organization of Resident Representatives who discuss issues pertinent to resident well-being.

Visit the websites of all the organizations listed above as they contain helpful, up-to-date information on well-being, learning, finances, and contractual issues, and provide hundreds of useful links of interest to residents. Your own national specialty association is likely to have a section for residents and fellows as well.

Setting Up Your Own Support Group

- Establish resident interest in attending a group and determine feasible frequency. Offer healthy food!
- Approach the program director for expertise, suggestions, and funding if a mental health professional is to lead the group. The

director's support is necessary, particularly if residents are to be
freed from their duties to attend.

- Decide whether the group is to be self-led or led by a non-
evaluating faculty member or mental health professional. Keep in
mind that most residents prefer to meet on their own and lead/
chair their own meetings.
- Plan logistics carefully. Aim for weekly or biweekly meetings lasting 45 to 60 minutes, possibly over lunch, and attended by seven to
10 people. Arrange coverage for those attending and provide food.
- Consider holding a resident retreat away from the hospital once or
twice a year.
- Prepare and publicize a list of resources for emergency healthcare
should members need outside help.
- Remember your goals: the group provides support, not psychotherapy. It will help members to air their feelings ("gripe sessions"),
normalize stresses, and solve problems. Topics can be chosen in
advance, or pressing concerns can guide the format of each meeting. The amount of self-revelation will vary, but the focus should
be on shared problem solving regarding residency stresses and on
physician–patient and physician–staff relations. Members should
speak for themselves, not for each other.
- Prepare a list of 10 to 12 difficult situations or scenarios that residents are likely to face in training (e.g., verbal abuse, arranging
organ donation, facing a clinical error).
- A good group leader will encourage but not teach or guide content,
and will defuse conflict and comment on process only if it impedes
members' giving mutual support. (The leader may be more active,
interpreting underlying conflicts, if the group is an experiential or
process one.)
- Speakers can be invited, and films shown. Topics for discussion can
include burnout, fatigue, the "difficult patient," resident competence versus fear of error and failure, the dying patient, bearing
bad news, handling staff conflict, ethical dilemmas, the impaired
resident, stress-management techniques, career and financial planning, balancing family life, and a review of local, provincial or state,
and national resources. See the list at the end of chapter 8 for films,
videos, and literature that will prompt discussion on physician
identity.

- Provide links to online support and/or social media, including Facebook, for residents and their spouses. Swap strategies with colleagues in Canada and the United States.

Family medicine faculty at the Oakland University William Beaumont School of Medicine created and assessed an innovative, popular lunchtime curriculum on Meaning in Medicine. Here is their list of topics, which you may want to use/adapt to your own setting:

A Sample Lunchtime Curriculum[14]

Discussion Topics for Postgraduate Years (PGY) 1 and 2

- Reflecting upon patients' perceptions of healthcare providers
- Stereotyping in patient care
- Finding renewal
- Being present in what you do
- Dealing with patient death
- Recognizing changes in empathy along the way
- Reflecting upon what advice would have been helpful as a PGY 1 in July
- Developing skills (courage) to be imperfect
- Learning how to reach out and be connected
- Focusing on importance of team work and collaboration during and after residency
- Establishing goals for wellness – both personally and professionally
- Avoiding/dealing with burnout
- Focusing on "Mindfulness" for providers and patients
- Creating strategies for improving teamwork and morale
- Using personal strengths to cope and to improve professional and personal life

Discussion Topics for PGY 2 and 3

- Managing difficult patients
- Ethical issues of patient care
- Educational goals
- Time management and office efficiency
- Work/life balance

- Leadership considerations in future practice
- Post-graduate plans/career transition
- Managing technology
- Board preparation
- Patient anecdotes
- Improvements in residency training
- Emotional responses to bad outcomes
- Lifestyle considerations in future practice

MAXIMIZING A PERSONAL SENSE OF CONTROL[15]

Tait Shanafelt has written powerful and moving pieces on finding meaning, balance, and personal satisfaction in medicine.[15] He encourages physicians to identify their personal and professional values in order to see how these mesh or conflict over time. He has compiled the following list of questions to help identify values:

Personal Values

1 What is my greatest priority in life? Have I been living my life in a way that demonstrates this?
2 Where am I most irreplaceable? At home? At the hospital? Elsewhere?
3 Do I have adequate balance between my personal and professional lives?
4 Am I asking more of my spouse and children than I should?
5 What kind of a legacy do I want to leave my children?
6 What person or activity have I been neglecting?
7 If I could relive the past year, what would I spend more time doing? What would I spend less time doing? What changes do I need to make to help this happen this year?
8 Why did I choose my profession? What do I like most about my job?
9 What would I like my life to be like in 10 years?
10 What do I fear?

Shanafelt encourages doctors to reflect on their answers and to rank important priorities, noting areas of conflict or incompatibility. He suggests that physicians identify the areas of their work that are the most meaningful and satisfying to them (teaching, research, patient care, palliative care, etc.) and to let those insights guide career plans. Similarly, acknowledging areas of weakness may lead to extra training, shared learning, improvement of skills, and reduced stress. Finally, individual wellness strategies should be prioritized throughout a medical career, as described elsewhere in this book. These include nurturing relationships, exploring spirituality, developing non-medical hobbies, traveling, ensuring adequate sleep, exercise, nutrition, medical care, and protecting time for reflection and personal reassessment.

Practical Tips for Keeping Control and Balance at Work

Be creative in getting the most out of your training *and* free time.

- Try to plan your rotation schedule, aiming to alternate between difficult and easy, in-and outpatient rotations. Submit your request to your residency director well in advance.
- Request a transparent call and holiday request system that all residents can access and verify. Take your holidays – they don't carry over into the next year!
- Find out the names and rotation schedules of good senior residents and attending physicians and try to arrange to work on their services.
- Obtain a list of hospital statutory holidays and request some long weekends off well in advance.
- Plan and schedule holiday time well in advance; it provides an important respite and should be used strategically.
- Choose hospital assignments that require less call or home call. If possible, live close to the hospital, thereby saving travel time and increasing sleep time.
- Keep track of all night calls, particularly weekend or statutory holiday calls, so that you can request compensation for extras if appropriate. Inform your residency director or housestaff representative of contractual abuses.

- Remember the seasonal nature of rotations and plan accordingly (e.g., the pediatric outpatient department is flat in the summer, and surgery is slow at Christmas).
- Maximize elective time by arranging interesting locations and subject matter. Do not be afraid to request something or somewhere original, and document all arrangements by letter.
- Pamper yourself when you are stressed (e.g., take a taxi, order out, hire a cleaner, buy yourself flowers, call long distance to a friend).
- Control your learning. Ask questions and request increased teaching, supervision, or lectures. Ask for one-on-one instruction if you need it.
- Be aware of all the benefits available to you through the hospital and university: library and sports facilities, legal and financial advisers, leaves of absence. Use allotted conference times to learn, explore new locations, and make valuable contacts. Professional, specialty, or society meetings are often inspiring.
- Sometimes crossing each day off on a calendar is a satisfying symbol of getting through. Buy a one-year calendar to record holidays and rotations. Note pay days, special occasions, and deadlines (e.g., references for jobs and exam applications).
- Plan your time every day, listing priorities and "scut" work and eliminating unnecessary tasks. Order consultations, tests, and support staff services (e.g., electrocardiograms and intravenous drips) early in the day when they are available. Save yourself travel time by developing a system for doing all work (e.g., X-rays) floor by floor or department by department. Make lists when you feel you are losing control, and note pros and cons and options. Consider keeping a journal, or jot down milestones or key events (like "first delivery," "first solo resuscitation") on your calendar for a personal record of your journey through residency.

TIP: "I recommend batching tasks if possible, e.g., reviewing all outstanding bloodwork and imaging at 10 pm if possible and deferring any non-urgent checks until, say, 6 AM."

- Make a list with your colleagues of "time drainers" on your service (disorganized sign-outs, lack of access to computers, delays contacting insurance companies) and problem-solve together to find and prioritize solutions. Make a list of your own "time wasters" and find solutions for each.

- Remember that you are entitled to sick days, which can be taken when you are feeling particularly under stress. Do not be irresponsible to resident colleagues or expect them to do your work, but consider taking a "mental health day," which will allow you to return rested and more effective. Find out if you are required to "work back" those days.
- Some programs tolerate leaves of absence lasting from 20 days to 3 months without penalty at the discretion of the residency program director. Find out to whom your leave will be reported (i.e., licensing bodies). Keep this option in mind if things get out of hand and discuss it with the director.
- Take rotation evaluations seriously and do not sign one that you disagree with. Request clarification or rewording rather than waiting for surprises; request regular feedback if you are not getting it during rotations.
- Periodically ask for access to your personnel file to verify its content and accuracy.
- Obtain a copy of your hospital or union contract and read it carefully. Know what is expected of you and what protection you can expect.
- Remember to keep your options open. Learn the requirements for a general license so that you can take outside work. Find out the varying provincial and state requirements for internship and residency, and keep copies of all correspondence should these requirements change.
- If you are disappointed or overwhelmed, you can attempt to change programs or hospital bases as other positions become vacant (check the specialty journals), sometimes even in mid-year.
- Don't complain and don't blame. Get political. Consider running for a position in your hospital, national, provincial, or state housestaff association; or as chief resident, faculty representative; regional representative to your specialty association; regional AMA resident physician representative in the United States; or representative to the university or to the university's committee on residency training.

- Find out about PHPs and physician well-being groups in your area. Talk to the hospital program director about setting up resident–staff feedback (or "gripe sessions"), a resident support group, or a resident peer review system in which residents participate in evaluating each other's progress and in selecting new candidates of the residency program. If you are a US trainee, and there is no union at your hospital, talk about starting one.
- Complete all professor and rotation evaluations. This is not a hopeless gesture but an important source of feedback for program change. If your program doesn't have them, develop the forms yourself. Be fair, honest, and don't complete them on a day when you're fed up![15]

PERSONAL STRATEGIES FOR MAINTAINING BALANCE

Check in with yourself on a regular basis. Are you happy? fulfilled? well-supported?

- As Shanafelt suggests, list your goals: professional, personal, romantic, family, financial, spiritual, physical, and so on. Decide to what degree you have attained some of them and what now prevents you from attaining others. Pay attention to your creative side and to how music, literature, and film relax you and enrich your interactions with and understanding of patients. (A medical humanities bibliography is provided in chapter 13.)
- Consider keeping a journal or writing narratives about your ward experiences as ways to promote self-reflection.
- Know and develop your personal coping skills. Chatting with others, humor, naps, hobbies, exercise, and leisure time help reduce stress. Determine which activities are most effective for you and build them into your schedule, even if it means sometimes saying "no" at home and at work.

TIP: "I think it is important to make a point of taking breaks on call. Even on a busy service, taking a few minutes to go to the washroom, close my eyes, breathe, play with my phone for a few minutes, makes me feel a lot better when I get back to work ten minutes later."

- Identify one interest or activity that grounds you outside of medicine, and make time for it every week.
- Reframe a tendency toward self-criticism by identifying one satisfying event or exchange every day. Remember: you know more today than you did yesterday. Try to live day to day, because you cannot delay gratification indefinitely.
- Try to have one meaningful conversation per day.
- Draw a self-esteem pie chart and indicate what portions currently represent work, love (relationships), play (hobbies/creativity), and spirituality. Post the diagram on your fridge next to what you would *like* your pie to look like if it were more balanced.

- Keep your home a safe refuge. Make it as comfortable as you can. Don't live in boxes!

REFERENCES

1 Rosen IM, Christie JD, Bellini LM, et al. Health and health care among housestaff in four U.S. internal medicine residency programs. *J Gen Intern Med.* 2000;15(2):116–21. http://dx.doi.org/10.1046/j.1525-1497.2000.11218.x.

2 Weidner BC, Dennis BM, Ayoub MM, et al. Addressing trainees' concerns through a resident advocacy committee. *Am Surg.* 2014;80(3):307–8.

3 Siegel B, Donnelly JC. Enriching personal and professional development: The experience of a support group for interns. *J Med Educ.* 1978;53:908–14.

4 Butler R. Support groups address residents' personal development. *JAMA.* 1993;93:789–91.

5 Weight CJ, Sellon JL, Lessard-Anderson CR, et al. Physical activity, quality of life, and burnout among physician trainees: The effect of a team-based, incentivized exercise program. *Mayo Clin Proc.* 2013;88(12):1435–42. http://dx.doi.org/10.1016/j.mayocp.2013.09.010.

6 Pliego JF, Wehbe-Janek H, Rajab MH, et al. Ob/gyn boot camp using high-fidelity human simulators: Enhancing residents' perceived competency, confidence in taking a leadership role, and stress hardiness. *Simul Healthc.* 2008;3(2):82–9. http://dx.doi.org/10.1097/SIH.0b013e3181658188.

7 Costello J, Livett M, Stride PJO, et al. The seamless transition from student to intern: From theory to practice. *Intern Med J.* 2010;40(10):728–31. http://dx.doi.org/10.1111/j.1445-5994.2010.02272.x.

8 Laack TO, Newman JS, Goyal DG, et al. A 1-week simulated internship course helps prepare medical students for transition to residency. *Simul Healthc.* 2010;5(3):127–32. http://dx.doi.org/10.1097/SIH.0b013e3181cd0679.

9 Bragard I, Etienne A, Merckaert I, et al. Efficacy of a communication and stress management training on medical residents' self-efficacy, stress to communicate and burnout. *J Health Psychol.* 2010;15(7):1075–81. http://dx.doi.org/10.1177/1359105310361992.

10 Satterfield JM, Becerra C. Developmental challenges, stressors and coping strategies in medical residents: A qualitative analysis of support groups. *Med Educ.* 2010;44(9):908–16. http://dx.doi.org/10.1111/j.1365-2923.2010.03736.x.

11 Levey RE. Sources of stress for residents and recommendations for programs to assist them. *Acad Med.* 2001;76(2):142–50. http://dx.doi.org/10.1097/00001888-200102000-00010.

12 Howell JB, Schroeder DP (eds). *Physician Stress: A Handbook for Coping.* Baltimore: University Park Press; 1984.

13 Shanafelt TD. Finding meaning, balance, and personal satisfaction in the practice of oncology. *J Support Oncol.* 2005;3:157–64.

14 Van Dyke A, Seger AM. Finding, keeping, and revitalizing the meaning in family medicine. *Int J Psychiatry Med.* 2013;45(4):323–31. http://dx.doi.org/10.2190/PM.45.4.c.

15 Beckman T, Reed D, Shanafelt TD. Impact of resident wellbeing and empathy on assessment of faculty physicians. *J Gen Intern Med.* 2010;25(1):52–6. http://dx.doi.org/10.1007/s11606-009-1152-0.

Protecting and Improving Personal Relationships

The people who thrive during residency are those who maintain friendships and family relationships and build new relationships as they go. As mentioned earlier, having a loving partner and supportive community are necessary ingredients of happiness for all human beings, and will also protect you from some of the effects of work stress. On the flipside, the busy schedule during residency may make it difficult for you to spend time with those you love. Here are some tips and strategies for doing so.

COUPLE LIFE

The stresses of training that tax residents particularly affect their couple life. Residents' lack of time, exhaustion, absence, and general unavailability often produce conflict at home. Because most residents' partners also work outside the home,[1] the scheduling of quality time and household duties is complex. Historically, wives of physicians score high on interpersonal sensitivity, depression, and hostility scales.[2] Husbands of physicians may feel threatened by their wives' success, level of responsibility, or income and decision-making power. In his book *Doctors' Marriages: A Look at the Problems and Their Solutions*,[3] Myers points out that the key stressors for the married resident often depend on the developmental level of the couple (e.g., newly married vs settled, childless vs with children).

Large educational debts, the increasingly uncertain future of some specialties, and moonlighting for extra cash at the expense of free time also make money a significant issue for couples.

October 1st, by Mairi Leining

You ask about my day –
I should have taken a Polaroid;
lime curtains, black sheets,
yellow man, your age,
rusted nails on restless fingers,
pregnant belly with twisted purple veins,
afraid to ask for directions.

Said he drank to escape the loneliness.
That down escalator, no basement floor.

I hold his hand, breathe through my mouth,
Discuss the facts from yesterday's spill;
a new liver, perhaps.

You ask about my day –
I tell you it was fine;
my side of the bed grows farther.

Moving to another city adds pressures to relationships. Residents find that getting started in their training program can give a stimulating and structured focus to relocating. Their partners, however, may feel ambivalent about the move and burdened by the logistics. They can feel isolated, and lonely for friends and family in the new city. They can sometimes feel like their career or personal aspirations come second. This can be especially true for the spouses of international medical graduates. Social life gradually diminishes because there is little time to see other couples or family members. The common-law, gay, other-race, or recently immigrated partner of a medical resident may feel particularly stigmatized in a conservative medical social milieu or general community. Some couples are geographically separated by the match and try to maintain long-distance relationships, which involve their own stressors.[4]

The resident's personality may change so much during training (e.g., with a tendency toward irritability, hypersensitivity, or overconfidence) that the partner may feel abandoned. Residents concerned about their career choice or competence may become more preoccupied and withdrawn, and they may shut out their partners because of feelings of shame and failed responsibility. The high levels of resident exhaustion can cause changes in the quality of a couple's sex life, which the partner may perceive as rejection. Partners may also believe that their concerns are dwarfed by those of physicians who are diligently saving lives and who have grown accustomed to adopting a direct and authoritative stance. Some residents even develop a psychiatric illness (see chapter 1), which may precipitate or aggravate conflict in the relationship.

TIP: "It may be good to spend a half-hour extra at the hospital tidying stuff up or doing non-clinical work (e.g., research) so that you can be fully devoted to home life at the end of the day."

Decisions that are usually shared, such as the timing of having children and settling versus moving, become more complicated for both partners, particularly for women physicians, who experience "role strain" (the wish to be "super" physicians, mothers, wives, and daughters). Household tasks and raising children often constitute the most frequent sources of resident couple conflict. Unfortunately, medical colleagues may not acknowledge the value of male residents' trying to reduce the risks of conflict by participating in these tasks. One recent study showed how stressed resident spouses were as compared to faculty spouses.[5]

Surviving Residency, a wonderful book written by Kristen Math, a medical spouse, has tips on moving, finding housing and schools for your children, and organizing finances.

AVOIDING TROUBLE IN COUPLE LIFE[6,7]

Here are some tips and considerations to help you avoid trouble in couple life:

- Remember that your partner is not medically trained and may need frequent explanations about expectations, scientific terms, causes of stress, procedures, and duties; however, avoid constant shop talk.
- Write out a schedule of shifts and rotations or online call

schedules with probable hours, so your partner knows what to expect. Make a list of household tasks with your partner and discuss how to share them, taking into account each other's workloads.

- Plan time alone together in advance, rather than hoping it will happen. Go out on a "date" at least once a week!
- Leave the job at the hospital. Avoid constant calls to the hospital or worrying about things you might have forgotten.
- If you're both doctors, try to book the same calls.
- Acknowledge when you are tired, angry, or sad, and state the source of the feeling (the job, home, or elsewhere).
- Set aside a regular time to talk about your priorities and long-term goals as a couple, emphasizing things to look forward to.
- Call, Skype, or text home at least once a shift.
- Do things to increase closeness: have dinner together at the hospital on a call night, telephone each other, leave notes, arrange surprises, buy gifts, make playful gestures.
- Develop shared hobbies and activities: sports, gardening, home improvement, family visits, and so forth.
- Maximize support from family, friends, social events, and residency resources.
- Schedule time for sex – because of fatigue levels, if you don't, it might not happen![8]

Signs Of Trouble In Couple Life[3]

When there is trouble in couple life, try to recognize it early. Here are some of the signs:

- Increased quarrelling, particularly over "picky" issues
- Decreased relating (talking, sex, leisure, play, or vacation time)
- Avoidance behaviors (like over-booking your personal schedule)
- Sexual infidelity
- Fear of "nothing left in common"
- Symptoms of anxiety, depression, or substance abuse in either or both partners
- Increased unresolved anger or anger exhibited passively or violently

TIP: *"I encourage my interns and students going home for the holidays to ask their family members and loved ones who are not in medicine what those people want in a doctor, and to reflect on whether that's what my trainees want to be; and to reflect on why or why not."*

Dealing with Conflict[3]

Couple life involves conflicts, not only in couples of which one or both are medical residents. The following are some ways of dealing with conflict:

- Label problems in a non-accusatory way.
- Use "we" rather than "you" in discussions.
- Separate internal (couple) issues from external ones (e.g., residency time pressures).
- Listen openly and avoid a defensive stance or attitude.
- Acknowledge that problems may be situational or temporary, but do not pretend they will simply disappear.
- Try to develop mutual support and support from family, friends, and other couples.
- Protect or add time for talking, play, sex, and vacations.
- Investigate options such as residency support groups, marriage retreats, and counseling through your religious community, resident services, wellness office, or the hospital department of psychiatry or psychology.
- If you are looking for a couples' counselor, the American Association for Marriage and Family Therapy lists therapists taking patients at www.therapistlocator.net. In Canada, ask your family doctor for a referral.

FRIENDS AND FAMILY

Social media (despite some of their professional drawbacks described later) in some ways make it easier to let people know you're thinking of them, chat, or make plans for when you are free. You can text, email, and Skype when you have a free moment with your smartphone or laptop. Be sure to ask family members how they're doing as they may be inclined to focus on you and on what they know of residency stress. Let your parents, grandparents, siblings, nieces and nephews, and god-children know that you love them, and that you haven't changed (or are not letting yourself change) when it comes to them.

Should You Medically Treat a Friend or Family Member?[9]

It's not unusual for family members to ask for medical advice and/or treatment. To avoid potential complications and the boundary blurring inherent in caring for family and friends, here are key questions to ask yourself before medically treating a friend or family member.

1 Does my relative's presenting problem fall into my area of exper-tise? Am I trained and/or equipped to deal with the problem?
2 Am I equipped to deal with a relative's personal or sexual history in an objective way? Could I deliver bad news or a poor prognosis honestly if required?
3 Am I objective enough not to defensively over-treat, or not to use denial regarding the severity of the problem and undertreat?
4 If I help a particular family member medically, what effect will this have on family conflicts, patterns, or dynamics?
5 Will my friend or family member do as I suggest (comply with treatment) or take advice less seriously because of the personal con-nection?
6 Will I, through anxiety or a sense of entitlement, interfere with care once my friend or family member is referred to a colleague?
7 Am I willing to be held accountable ethically and medicolegally if my care is judged substandard, incomplete, or inadequate?

Generally, with the exception of emergencies, it is preferable to refer a family member to a colleague. Refer to the state or provincial associa-tion for specific guidelines. They usually discourage or forbid treating/prescribing for family and close friends.

PARENTING

This section is addressed principally to all residents and may be of par-ticular use for female residents; however, their partners and other sup-portive colleagues who share the responsibilities of parenting should learn to appreciate the importance of the issues and the suggestions they present. Happily, male residents are increasingly making use of paternity leave as well.

- Let go of perfection! As the famous child psychoanalyst D.W. Winnicott said to parents, you just have to be "good enough."
- During parental leave, keep up to date by reading journals in your specialty and consider the rewards of returning to work you do well; do not view your return to residency as the enemy.
- Investigate child care options (day care, in-home babysitting, or live-in help).
- Given irregular work schedules and the frequency of childhood illnesses, remember the need for backup; day care centers tend to have fixed drop-off and pick-up times. When hiring at-home help, interview applicants with your partner and check all references. Look for someone with a flexible attitude toward duties (including cooking and light housekeeping), availability, and hours; procedures on rotations and rounds will make the timing of your arrival home unpredictable. Before you finish your maternity leave, arrange to observe how candidates interact with your child. Do not scrimp or rush when hiring a caregiver with whom your child will form a significant bond. You must be satisfied that the relationship will be a good one.
- Remember that a portion of child care costs is tax creditable; keep receipts.
- Because residency hours tend to be inflexible, flexibility at home is important. Discuss and agree with your partner on how to share the parenting responsibilities, and try to arrange elective rotations with flexible hours for your return after maternity leave.
- Ask your attending physician to finish rounds at a reasonable hour and arrange coverage with another resident for emergencies.
- For family emergencies, recruit other support for your role as a parent among friends, neighbors, family, and in-laws by asking them to help and to visit your child regularly.
- Ask colleagues with children for other strategies.

- Be available on your cellphone so that your caregiver can reach you in emergencies (you will feel more comfortable knowing that you are available) and call home or Skype every day to say "Hi" to older children.
- Establish regular rituals with your children to ensure you spend quality time with them; when you come home tired at the end of the day, for example, try a 5-minute cuddle session. Set a time that follows your own rest period for playing or reading stories.
- Make your "off-call" time inviolate for your family; plan holiday time in advance, even if you stay home, so that the whole family has something to look forward to.
- Try to do your reading at work, because it will be next to impossible to do it at home.
- Avoid a tendency to reproach yourself for not being the ideal parent-physician. You and your family *will* survive the rigors of residency!

Other Parenting Resources

Lobby for daycare/childcare resources and subsidies.[10,11] The following resources will assist you in exploring options and decision making as a working parent:

- American Academy of Pediatrics: https://www.aap.org/en-us/Pages/Default.aspx
  Includes suggested professional resources:
  http://pediatriccare.solutions.aap.org/Pediatric-Care.aspx
  https://brightfutures.aap.org/
- J Bickel, *Medicine and Parenting: A Resource for Medical Students, Residents, Faculty and Program Directors* (AAMC, Washington, DC – https://www.aamc.org)
- Other resources:
  http://residentdoctorsbc.cawp-content/uploads/2010/12/Parenting-Guide-2014_pages.pdf

http://www.cjem-online.ca/v4/n4/ (article about issues becoming
a parent during residency)
http://www.aafp.org/about/policies/all/parental-leave.html
- Your residency well-being office may offer parenting workshops. If
not, ask for them!

THE SINGLE RESIDENT

Medical residents who are single and live alone may be at increased
emotional risk because of a lack of support mechanisms; they may
become increasingly isolated socially because they have little time or
energy to meet new people or to date. They may also be reluctant to
acknowledge feelings of loneliness to themselves or others because
such feelings are not part of their self-concept as competent professionals. Most of their initial social contacts come from the hospital, because
they are often in a new city, and their schedule tends to keep them from
exploring. For some residents, this is not a happy prospect.

Coping Mechanisms for Single Residents

- Remember your need for support from family and friends
throughout residency, and avoid the tendency to withdraw
socially when fatigued or to deny feelings of loneliness.
- Attend hospital social events, especially at the beginning of
residency. You have to start socializing sometime, and you will
meet other, non-hospital-affiliated people at these occasions.
- Make it a rule not to talk shop with medical friends at social
occasions. Cultivate nonmedical friends through sports, hobbies, or religious groups.
- If you live alone, equip your land line or cell phone to take
messages, so that you do not miss invitations.
- Use social media judiciously to date, make friends, and build
a community. Remember that posts and pictures are there
forever!

- Consider joining a health club, a religious group, your build-ing's tenants' association, or special-interest or political groups, realizing, however, that you may have to miss some meetings.
- Make yourself go out socially, even if you're tired.
- Consider living with a compatible medical or nonmedical roommate. Establish clear rules about quiet time (post-call), sharing chores, and so on.
- Schedule vacations with friends well in advance so that you have something to look forward to.
- Request your call nights well in advance so that you can plan your social life (e.g., special concerts and long weekends away).
- Maintain links with family members, even if they live in another city, through visits, frequent telephone calls, texting, and e-mail.

Should You Date a Patient?[12]

In today's medicolegal environment, socializing with patients may be ill advised because of accusations of boundary violations.

Here are some suggested guidelines regarding romantic or sexual involvement with a patient. Check with your local medical professional association or licensing body for up-to-date local recommendations.

- Sexual relationships between patients in active (current) treatment and doctors must be avoided.
- A period of time (usually one year) should lapse between the date of the last medical follow-up with the patient and the onset of the romantic or sexual contact.
- Where treatment has involved psychoanalysis, psychotherapy, or extensive counseling, sexual or romantic involvement with the patient should be avoided (and is prohibited by many professional associations).
- Special caution should be exercised before a physician starts dating a former patient if the professional context with the patient resulted in the patient's emotional dependency on the doctor or created any other vulnerability that may have impaired the patient's judgment or ability to make free decisions.

- Pay attention to how long you've known the patient, what care you've provided, and other relevant circumstances before dating. If in doubt, consult an impartial colleague or psychotherapist.
- Your local college or licensing body will also have statements on this matter.

REFERENCES

1 Landau C, Hall S, Wartman SA, et al. Stress in social and family relationships during the medical residency. *J Med Educ.* 1986;61:654–60.
2 Smith MF, Andrasik F, Quinn SJ. Stressors and psychological symptoms of family practice residents and spouses. *J Med Educ.* 1988;63:397–405.
3 Myers M. *Doctors' Marriages: A Look at the Problems and Their Solutions.* New York: Plenum; 1988. http://dx.doi.org/10.1007/978-1-4684-9957-5.
4 Guldner GT. Long-distance relationships and emergency medicine residency. *Ann Emerg Med.* 2001;37(1):103–6. http://dx.doi.org/10.1067/mem.2001.371103.
5 Sargent MC, Sotile W, Sotile MO, et al. Quality of life during orthopaedic training and academic practice: Part 2: spouses and significant others. *J Bone Joint Surg Am.* 2012;94(19):e145 1. http://dx.doi.org/10.2106/JBJS.K.00991.
6 Jaco JM. *Can We Live with This Job?* Toronto: PAIRO; 1989.
7 Myers M. Medical marriages and other intimate relationships. *Medical Journal of Australia* 2002;181392–3.
8 Sangi-Haghpeykar H, Ambani DS, Carson SA. Stress, workload, sexual well-being and quality of life among physician residents in training. *Int J Clin Pract.* 2009;63(3):462–7. http://dx.doi.org/10.1111/j.1742-1241.2008.01845.x.
9 La Puma J, Preist E. Is there a doctor in the house? An analysis of the practice of physicians treating their own families. *JAMA.* 1992;267(13):1810–2. http://dx.doi.org/10.1001/jama.1992.03480130126037.
10 Key LL Jr. Child care supplementation: Aid for residents and advantages for residency programs. *J Pediatr.* 2008;153(4):449–50. http://dx.doi.org/10.1016/j.jpeds.2008.05.028.
11 Hurt A. Family matters. *The New Physician*, March 2010. http://www.amsa.org/404.
12 Dempsey L, Ecker J. Understanding the dating guidelines. *CPSO Members' Dialogues*, Nov. 1994; 9–11.

CHAPTER SIX

Keeping Professional Relationships Healthy

Let's face it. You'll be spending more time with fellow residents and supervisors than anybody else for the next few years. If you're lucky, you'll be part of a functional, caring team. Your team may start that way then deteriorate or be dysfunctional from the get-go. Here are some tips on avoiding trouble.

Impaired housestaff team relations usually go undetected by staff supervisors and are usually not addressed by residents themselves. The results are increased anxiety for team members and, ultimately, compromised patient care. The varieties of resident personalities and associated interactive styles significantly affect the development of housestaff teams, as does the tendency of residents to hide worries from each other in an attempt to appear competent. Attending physicians may be absent most of the time, and senior or chief residents may be unaccustomed to a leadership and teaching role or more interested in exploiting their new position in the hospital hierarchy to reduce their own workload. Conflict is not defused in such circumstances.

One way to avoid conflict is to spell out roles, duties, and expectations at the start of a rotation (see tables 6.1 and 6.2).

Table 6.1 Know Your Roles

Year	Responsibilities	Key Role
Intern(e)	Initial patient evaluation Routine patient care decisions Organize patients' care	Apprentice Junior teacher
Junior resident	Supervise interns and students Approve diagnosis and management Demonstrate ability to work with other personnel	Team supervisor Teaching role expected Troubleshooter for minor conflicts Key person for attending physician
Senior resident	Competent team supervision Able to handle complex patients	Senior advisor for junior residents Conflict resolution of more significant issues Competent team teacher
Attending Physician	Assures team can handle essential concepts of medicine Stimulates reading on core materials Reviews charts and orders for completeness	Teacher Mentor Handle major conflicts

Source: Adapted from Alguire P, Whelan G, Rajput V, *The International Medical Graduate's Guide to US Medicine & Residency Training*, Philadelphia: ACP Press; 2009.

Table 6.2 Know Your Responsibilities

Your Responsibilities

1 Admit new patients
2 Visit and examine all patients on your team each morning
3 Attend work rounds
4 Present your case, update chart notes
5 Teach medical students
6 Communicate with other care-team members
7 Order appropriate labs and imaging studies
8 Order appropriate and early consultations
9 Attend follow-up and sign-out rounds
10 Plan discharge and dictate discharge note
11 Arrange discharge meds
12 Educate patient regarding discharge instructions and arrange follow-up

Source: Adapted from Alguire P, Whelan G, Rajput V, *The International Medical Graduate's Guide to US Medicine & Residency Training*, Philadelphia: ACP Press; 2009.

SIGNS OF TROUBLE AMONG RESIDENTS[1]

Where there is trouble among residents, there is also likely to be:

- Increased sarcasm
- Increased petty disagreements over esoteric points
- Formation of factions and scapegoating
- Increased sick leave, lateness, and longer rounds
- Decreased morale and increased anger, depression, and fatigue in team members
- Decreased attendance and helpfulness in teaching and coverage
- Power struggles (e.g., changing others' orders)
- Unfinished work (a risk to patients)

TIP: *"I think it is important to get to know about the other members on a team ASAP. E.g., their life before and outside of medicine; their aspirations within medicine; their strengths and weaknesses as they identify them; and what they think about other members of the team (to identify problem spots earlier)."*

DEALING WITH TEAM TROUBLES

When there is trouble among residents, deal with it using the following strategies:

- Define the problem (e.g., external stress or interpersonal tension).
- Arrange an initial team meeting to let off steam ("gripe sessions").
- Keep the discussion "team-" or "we-" oriented rather than accusing people. Talk about behaviors, not personalities.
- If the initial meeting is unsuccessful, recruit the attending physician, senior resident, or a hospital mediator to intervene.

Preventing Conflict

Best of all, however, is trying to prevent conflict in the first place. Here are some tips for preventing conflict among residents:

- Define roles in each new team (see table 6.1).
- Don't be late for meetings.

- Schedule informal rounds over lunch or pizza.
- Encourage team support by acknowledging shared moments of stress and anxiety.
- Schedule prophylactic mid-rotation "gripe sessions" for stressful rotations (e.g., in intensive care or surgery). Keep lines of communication open!
- Show each other courtesy and respect. Don't text/web-surf when someone is giving a talk or speaking at a meeting.
- Introduce appropriate humor to rounds.
- Consider arranging occasional dinners or social meetings outside the hospital.
- Work on your own leadership skills.
- Request that your program arrange annual day-long or weekend wellness retreats.

HOW TO BE AN EMOTIONALLY INTELLIGENT TEAM MEMBER

Business leaders remind us how to exhibit high EQ on the job:

- Be able to identify and name your feelings.
- Stay curious about co-workers.
- Embrace change.
- Identify your own strengths and weaknesses.
- Don't take things personally or get offended easily!
- Try to read people fairly but shorten/avoid/neutralize toxic encounters.
- Don't be a perfectionist and forgive others for their mistakes. Let go of grudges.
- Be assertive – learn how to say "no."
- Be grateful for what you have and generous with others.
- Challenge negative self-talk when it occurs. Stick with the evidence about how you're really doing.

(Source: www.entrepreneur.com)

Often conflict between residents on different teams or services occurs because of unclear requests or expectations, "turf wars," or patient "dumping," when one team wants to transfer care. Here are some suggestions for effective consulting and liaison.

AVOIDING TURF WARS: 10 COMMANDMENTS FOR EFFECTIVE CONSULTATION[2]

These tips are from a classic paper from the 1980s, but the rules hold up today.

1 Determine the real consultation question – call the consultee when necessary.
2 Establish urgency – emergent, urgent, or routine.
3 Look for yourself – examine the patient, review old data, and collect new information. Summarize lab/key test data for yourself.
4 Be as brief as appropriate – there is no need to repeat in full detail the data already recorded in the chart. Provide a primary and differential diagnosis.
5 Be specific, brief, and goal-oriented regarding treatment recommendations.
6 Provide a prognosis and contingency plans – anticipate potential problems. Offer a "decision tree" for problem solving.
7 Honor thy turf – don't take over the patient's care, unless requested to do so. Increasingly, specialists and family doctors are "sharing care" in an ongoing fashion.
8 Teach with tact – give references and communicate important information courteously and personally.
9 Provide direct personal contact – introduce yourself to the team members when you arrive on the ward and tell them how to get in touch with you, especially if your recommendations are crucial or potentially controversial.
10 Follow up – provide suggestions for follow-up in the hospital and make suggestions for arranging outpatient care.

THE IMPAIRED COLLEAGUE

How to deal with a colleague who is impaired poses a serious medical and ethical dilemma for physicians who feel torn between protecting a friend or colleague and protecting the patients that person serves. First, how do you distinguish between stress and impairment? Signs of impairment, addiction, or burnout that exceed the intermittent symptoms of fatigue include the following:

- Unexplained lateness and absence
- Carelessness, indifference, apathy, and increased mistakes in patient care
- Visible drug or alcohol abuse; pervasive clinical symptoms of anxiety, depression, psychosis (paranoia), mania, impaired memory, talk of suicide, and hopelessness
- Increased preoccupation with marital or professional conflicts
- Decreased efficiency (unfinished work, sometimes despite longer hours)
- More frequent angry outbursts
- Physical deterioration: weight loss or diminished grooming
- Other marked personality changes
- Patient complaints about a physician's attitudes or demeanor

Signs of alcohol and/or substance abuse include the following:

- Personality changes: increased anxiety, mood swings, decreased efficiency/reliability/decisiveness
- Increased absenteeism
- Increased reports of drug "loss," "wastage," or "spoilage"
- Visible intoxication on the job; alcohol on the breath
- Individual insists on working alone
- Individual insists on wearing long sleeves (to hide needle tracks) or disappears frequently (e.g., "to the washroom")
- Inappropriate affect, behavior, comments

There are several ways of handling impaired colleagues. If they pose no immediate risk to themselves or to patients:

- State your concern in a gentle, private, and non-accusatory fashion – patient safety comes first. If possible, balance this with a positive comment ("You've always been a good physician, and I'm worried about you"). "The non-coercive approach, with the possibility of punishment or coercion in the background, has been shown to be most successful."[3]

- State your personal observations and those of others, so that denial can be reduced.
- Ask for the individual's view of the problem.
- Give the individual information on how to contact residents' professional associations that provide confidential help and ask her to tell you later what she has done. Offer to arrange an evaluation with a caregiver; do not take on the treatment yourself.
- Warn the individual that if you do not receive any feedback, or if the problem worsens, you will be obliged to discuss the matter confidentially with your residency director. (You may wish to do this first if you feel unable to confront the resident yourself.) Policies about reporting impaired physicians vary; reporting may be obligatory in your area.
- Point out that obtaining help does not have to result in suspension, loss of income, or expensive treatment, but that delay might.
- Offer to attend the first assessment with the individual or encourage her to bring along someone close to her.

If they pose an immediate risk to themselves: Accompany them to the emergency department or call the psychiatrist on duty in your hospital. Do not leave them alone. Consider calling your provincial or state residents' association hotline where available.

If they pose an immediate risk to patients (e.g., are intoxicated before a delivery or a shift in the operating room or emergency department): Confront them discreetly with their current inability to perform. Offer to cover for them or to find coverage through the chief resident. If they refuse, call your attending physician immediately and inform your residency director. Patient safety is your priority.

Fortunately, programs like the JFK Family Practice Residency at the Robert Wood Johnson Medical School have written of their successes in working with impaired residents, demonstrating that intervention is well worth the effort. Consult the article by Winter and Birnberg[4] for a helpful algorithm on graded interventions that has proved helpful in such cases. (See the resources list in chapter 13 for treatment/referral information.) Nowadays, remedial programs available at PHPs are sophisticated and non-judgmental, and success rates are high, so early intervention is key.

RESIDENTS AS TEACHERS: WORKING WITH STUDENTS

All physicians remember particularly good or bad residents in their training whose actions and characteristics strongly influenced their choice of specialties. Being role models and teachers for students adds a further stress to residents' professional lives. (See chapter 8 for specific teaching strategies and resources.) No one has taught them how to teach, so they must learn by doing and from observing good and bad examples. Interviews conducted by this author with residents indicate that a good resident teacher:

- "Provided orientation when we arrived"
- Is accessible physically ("answers pages quickly") and emotionally ("doesn't make you feel stupid")
- Is connected and involved
- Has a good sense of humor and a capacity for making learning fun ("not overly anxious or compulsive")
- Is efficient ("keeps rounds short") and punctual
- Is practical ("simplifies things," "avoids esoteric emphasis")

TIP: *"I encourage my trainees to take notes on what they like and dislike about their senior residents. I like to say that I wrote all these things down and then when I became a senior resident, I did all the things I liked and avoided all the things I disliked, so that I only made mistakes I hadn't seen before."*

- Frequently gives positive feedback and patiently points out errors in patient care
- Stands up to the attending physician when necessary ("makes own decisions")
- Appears caring and conscientious and has good relations with patients and nurses
- Is fair (e.g., "about call duty")
- Is available for one-on-one teaching
- Knows how to handle team or interdisciplinary conflicts
- Does not foster excessive competition
- Is open to feedback
- Delegates responsibility appropriately

TIP: "Senior residents should ask patients: 'Who is the person most responsible for your care? What do you think about them?' I take notes and feed this back to my trainees and attendings."

- Demonstrates appropriate use of investigations and consultation
- Carries his own share of the workload
- Remembers what it was like to be a student or junior
- Creates a relaxed environment
- Is willing to teach hands-on procedures and assign level-appropriate tasks (read JC Edwards and RL Marier, *Clinical Teaching for Medical Residents: Roles*[5] and EH Morrison, "Yesterday a learner, today a teacher too"[6])

Remember to take your role as teacher seriously. Queen's University in Canada has produced guidelines for ethical teaching, excerpted below, which will help you reflect on your role as a teacher and may help launch discussion among residents and attending staff.[7]

If you identify that a student is struggling, it's best to identify them early and strategize discreetly with your attending staff and educational consultants if available at your hospital.[8]

Guide to the Ethical Behavior of Clinical Teachers[7]

The following are principles of ethical behavior for all clinical teachers, including those who may not be engaged directly in clinical practice.

1 Consider first the well-being of the patient.
2 Honor your profession and its traditions.
3 Recognize your limitations and the special skills of others in the prevention and treatment of disease.
4 Protect the patient's secrets (confidences).
5 Teach and be taught.
6 Remember that integrity and professional ability should be your best advertisement.
7 Be responsible in setting a value on your services.

Table 6.3 Overall Principles of Postgraduate Medical Education

---

1 Safe and effective care of the patient takes priority over the training endeavor.

2 Proper training optimizes patient care as well as the educational experience.

3 The autonomy and personal dignity of trainees and patients must be respected.

4 Joint decision-making and exchange of information between most responsible physician (i.e., the MD with final accountability for that patient), supervisor, and trainee provides an optimal educational experience.

5 Professionalism, which includes demonstration of compassion, service, altruism, and trustworthiness, is essential in all interactions in the training environment in order to provide the best quality care to patients.

Source: CPSO Policy Statement #2–11 – Professional Responsibilities in Postgraduate Medical Education, *Dialogue* 2011;2:2–3

Responsibilities to Students[7]

"Student" means any person involved in undergraduate or postgraduate healthcare training. The ethical clinical teacher is someone who:

- Will treat students with respect regardless of their level of training, race, creed, color, gender, sexual orientation, or field of study
- Will teach the knowledge, skills, attitudes, and behaviors, and provide the experience, that the student requires to become a physician in her chosen career
- Will supervise students at all levels of training as appropriate to their knowledge, skills, and experience
- Will support and encourage students in their endeavors to learn and to develop their skills and attitudes and a sense of enquiry
- Will allow responsibility commensurate with ability
- Will see patients when so requested by students
- Will teach students the rationale for decisions, the reasons for conclusions, the reasoning behind investigation and treatment
- Will discuss alternate diagnoses, investigations, and therapeutic choices and the merits and risks of these
- Will assess carefully and accurately students' abilities and provide prompt verbal and written feedback
- Will assess only performance and not allow assessment to be colored by personal interactions
- Will provide remedial teaching when so indicated by assessment

- Will maintain a professional teacher–student relationship at all times and avoid the development of emotional, sexual, financial, or other relationships with students
- Will strive to conduct herself in a fashion to be an excellent role model for students
- Will refrain from addressing students in a disparaging fashion
- Will refrain from intimidating or attempting to intimidate students
- Will refrain from harassment of students in any fashion – emotional, physical, or sexual

The Hotseat, by Richard M. Berlin

I swear by Apollo the physician, and Aesculapius, and Hygeia and Panacea, and all the gods and goddesses … to reckon him who taught me this Art equally clear to me as my parents …

– From the Hippocratic Oath

0700 and thirty housestaff collapse
like shipwreck survivors.
after 24 sleepless hours
of children renounced by Hygeia,
our eyes are drowned in shadow.
A few nod before he enters
ruddy-faced and rested, white coat starched and spotless:
Dr. Harry, Chief of the Mecca,
diagnostic wizard, the power
who can crush careers with a word.
He slaps a chest film on the light box
and hooks a bleary intern:
Tell me, doctor,
What is the shape of this child's ears?
Fifteen seconds, thirty, a minute of silence,
sweat weeps from the intern's forehead.
Harry scorches him with questions
and solves the riddle like Aesculpaius,
even kneads the intern's shoulders
as if soothing a bruise.
We curse him all day, stay awake

all night to earn his love,
and when we descend to Radiology
with our own tame students, we slap
a film on the light box and raise
their first beads of sweat.

BEING A TEAM PLAYER

Good relationships with nursing and other staff including physicians'
assistants, midwives, ward clerks, pharmacists, social workers, OTs/
PTs, and emergency medical technicians can make or break a residency
experience, given a resident's high daily level of contact with them. The
resident who feels threatened by competent nurses or physicians' assistants, and who feels superior or is sexist in interactions with others will
be labeled early in training and will find it difficult to achieve the level
of teamwork and camaraderie needed in the modern treating context.

To facilitate a good working relationship with nursing and other professional staff:

- Introduce yourself to all the nurses on your service when you begin
  to work there. If you find it congenial, give them permission to use
  your first name. Remember their names as well.
- Ask them for their opinions, and take their suggestions seriously.
  They may know the patient better than you do.
- Respect ward protocol and routines about orders, scheduling tests,
  and so on.
- Admit errors, including your own, and point out nursing errors in a
  private, non-accusatory, non-humiliating way.
- Do not show off or pull rank. Remember, you are working with fel-
  low professionals.
- Do not bluff if you do not know something. Say that you will find
  out.
- Use appropriate humor. Avoid sexist or flirtatious remarks and
  behavior.
- Try to develop a rapport with the head nurse, who may be a source
  of teaching and resource information and support.
- Be courteous and polite; say "please" and "thank you."

- Keep disputes patient-oriented; do not let them become personal.
- Request interprofessional education seminars to enhance shared learning and teamwork. Try to find out more about what your colleagues believe and actually do in their work lives.
- Communicate clearly.
- Provide information that is adequate and timely.
- Review nursing and other care-team notes before expressing your opinion.
- Document your communication with colleagues from other disciplines.
- One useful acronym for systematically structuring telephone calls about patients is DRAW: i.e., clearly articulating Diagnosis, Recent changes, Anticipated changes, and What to watch for.[9]

Beyond a discussion of "collegial relationships," there is an increasing emphasis on interprofessional education which encompasses optimal communication, collaboration, and conflict management among multiple healthcare professions and within teams. A detailed schematic framework for such learning is provided at www.ipe.utoronto.ca.

What is interprofessional education? The World Health Organization in 2010 defined it as follows: "Interprofessional education occurs when students from two or more professions learn about, from, and with each other to enable effective collaboration and improve health outcomes." Traditionally, medical students and residents have received teaching from their own discipline/profession, in order to master a specific body of shared medical knowledge, skills, and modes of conduct. Nowadays, almost all clinical settings involve teamwork among several professions. Students from various professions now learn together as a team. This allows for members to understand the core principle and concepts of each clinical discipline and to be familiar with the language and mindsets of those disciplines. (Source: www.ipe.utoronto.ca.)

Successful teamwork involves finding out what our colleagues believe, value, and do in their approach to patient care. A resident with good interprofessional skills can communicate clearly, effectively, and fairly, advocate for both patients and colleagues, recognize conflict and power differentials, and analyze personal values and professional beliefs (and entitlements) in an ongoing fashion.

The following questions can be helpful in understanding and improving team and group interactions during case conferences, team interventions, and seminars, and over the duration of specific rotations.

1 What professions are represented in this group?
2 How were different perspectives, communication styles, approaches represented in this rotation or educational seminar?
3 How does your professional training and/or professional lens inform your views and responses?
4 What similarities/differences have you observed among the different professions you have collaborated with? How do these relate to your own profession's values and roles in patient/client care?
5 How does the content in this discussion, case conference, or seminar reflect (or downplay) teamwork?
6 How can the different skill sets discussed be brought together to enhance the team response to patient care?
7 What have you learned and how well will this form your future work with colleagues of different disciplines?
8 Was the communication appropriate and equitable with respect to the information being exchanged by those present?
9 How well did your group members listen to each other?
10 How did you and others encourage collaboration as the group responded to new learning experiences? Who got left out?

ATTENDING PHYSICIANS

Residents are in a unique and sometimes awkward position because they are hospital employees, student apprentices, and responsible physicians all at the same time. The attending physician ("staffman") is both a type of boss who does not pay or hire residents and a teacher who evaluates residents' performance and has considerable power over their future. Overall, clinical skills, personality, and teaching ability are what residents identify as factors in selecting a staff physician as a role model. One study shows that five types of issues affect the relationship between supervisor and trainee: (1) compatibility of goals, (2) communication and feedback, (3) power and rivalry, (4) support and collegiality, and (5) level of expertise of both parties.[4] As residents' hours have become regulated, some staff doctors have grown resentful, assuming that "young doctors aren't as dedicated" or "are just in it for the lifestyle." Thus, an intergenerational clash of expectations can emerge. Attending physicians vary in their approaches, just as senior residents do; some have an interest in teaching and interacting with their housestaff, whereas others are remote or absent, and merely bill for residents' services. The concept of "medical student abuse" (either emotional or physical and sexual) applies equally to residents, who are particularly vulnerable because they need good evaluations to finish their training.

TIP: "I have found it very effective to meet with attendings before I work with them to get a sense of their styles and how they perceive their roles and the role of my team, and to make my own goals for the rotation clear."

Signs of Trouble in Resident–Attending Physician Relationship

The following are signs that there is trouble in the relationship between the medical resident and the attending physician:

- Sarcasm, harsh or hurtful criticism, verbal abuse, scapegoating (the target is usually a resident, who may complain covertly)
- Lack of positive feedback
- Racist, sexist, or other negative personal remarks directed at a resident
- Physical abuse (e.g., scalpel throwing, sexual advances)
- Decreased availability of the attending physician (late or absent for supervision, teaching, or rounds)
- Covering up attending physician's mistakes or unethical behavior
- Increased resident anxiety in the context of supervision by the attending physician
- Perception of the attending physician as incompetent, impaired, or unjust

- Feeling that evaluations are unfair
- Ceasing to care about work ("decathecting") because of an inability to please the attending physician

TIP: *"As a general rule, I think criticism should be private and praise should be public, and team members should NEVER be criticized in front of a patient."*

The following are signs of unprofessionalism in colleagues, as identified by the American Board of Internal Medicine (www.abim.org):

- Unmet professional responsibility
- Needs continual reminders about fulfilling responsibilities to patients and to other healthcare professionals
- Cannot be relied on to complete tasks
- Misrepresents or falsifies actions and/or information, for example, regarding patients, laboratory tests, research data
- Lack of effort toward self-improvement and adaptability
- Is resistant or defensive in accepting criticism
- Remains unaware of own inadequacies
- Resists considering or making changes
- Does not accept responsibility for errors or failure
- Is overly critical and/or verbally abusive during times of stress
- Demonstrates arrogance
- Diminished relationships with patients and families
- Lacks empathy and is often insensitive to patients' needs, feelings, and wishes or to those of the family
- Lacks rapport with patients and families
- Displays inadequate commitment to honoring the wishes and wants of the patient
- Diminished relationships with healthcare professionals
- Demonstrates inability to function within a healthcare team
- Lacks sensitivity to the needs, feelings, and wishes of the healthcare team

DEALING WITH UNPROFESSIONAL OR DISRUPTIVE BEHAVIOR BY RESIDENTS/ FACULTY

- Try to express your concerns privately.
- If you need to discuss your concerns with others, confide carefully and selectively to avoid gossip.
- Do not expose confidential issues in rounds or in front of colleagues.
- If you are acutely upset, excuse yourself briefly. Retain your composure, dignity, and professionalism. Do not retaliate and thereby lose your credibility.
- Document incidents, noting witnesses if necessary.
- Do not sign an evaluation that you think is unfair. If you disagree with it, appeal the evaluation according to established procedures.
- If you are injured or sexually harassed, check your contract and report the incident to the residency program director and consider legal action.
- If these measures do not resolve the problem, consult the residency program director about mediation or change of service or hospital.
- If there is still no resolution, contact the following (according to the increasing severity of the problem): the university department head and/or director of postgraduate education; the university harassment officer; the housestaff union lawyer; or the Resident Representative Committees at the Royal College of Physicians and Surgeons of Canada, or the American Medical Association in the United States.
- Demonstrate professional behavior yourself when introducing the issue.
- Know the policies at your school, program, and institution.
- Gather evidence/data.
- Know when you're in over your head – contact your housestaff association for advice.
- Contact your state/provincial housestaff and/or postgraduate officer, who will have guidelines on dealing with workplace intimidation/harassment/abuse.

- www.physicianhealth.com has excellent learning modules on the disruptive physician, as does the College of Physicians and Surgeons of Ontario: http://www.cpso.on.ca/CPSO/media/upload edfiles/policies/policies/Disruptive_Behaviour_Guidebook.pdf

HUMANISM AND PATIENT-CENTERED CARE: HOW TO BE A MINDFUL, CARING DOCTOR

A critique of modern medicine has been that evidence-based medicine favors population health, universal trends, and commonalities, rather than the uniqueness of a patient's experience of illness and the perceptions of his or her family members. This can lead to a physician-centered, hospital-centered, and disease-centered approach to illness and does not assist the patient with making meaning of their experiences with suffering.

Optimal Patient Care

The Institute of Medicine published *Crossing the Quality Chasm: A New Health System for the 21st Century* in the hopes of framing the emerging discussions on quality healthcare. Care should be:

1 Safe – care should be as safe for patients in healthcare facilities as in their homes.
2 Effective – the science and evidence behind healthcare should be applied and service standards maintained in the delivery of care.
3 Efficient – caring service should be cost-effective, and waste of equipment, supplies, ideas, and energy should be removed from the system.
4 Timely – the patient should experience no waits or delays in receiving care and service.
5 Equitable – unequal treatment should be a thing of the past. Disparity in care should be eradicated regardless of gender, ethnicity, geographic location, and socioeconomic status.
6 Patient-centered – the system of care should evolve around the patient, respect patient preferences, and put the patient in control.

Patient-centred care can be achieved by:

1 Exploring the patient's reason for visiting, their concerns, and their need for supportive information.
2 Providing an integrated understanding of the patient's world, understanding that there is a whole person with emotional needs and life issues, changes, and losses.
3 Finding common ground regarding what the problem is and mutually agreeing on its management
4 Enhancing prevention and health promotion and the continuing relationship between the patient, the doctor, and the patient's family and supports.

(Source: http://iom.nationalacademies.org)

In keeping with the goals of patient-centered care, Medical Humanism can be defined as "the fostering of relationships with patients that are empathic, compassionate, and include behaviors and attitudes that are sensitive to the person's values, autonomy, dignity, and cultural and ethnic backgrounds." The medical humanism movement seeks to understand the patient as a complete person with individual values, goals, and preferences with respect to clinical care and definitions of wellness.

The Arnold P. Gold Foundation (http://humanism-in-medicine.org) funds and promotes initiatives for improving patient care, and states: "Humanism in healthcare is characterized by a respectful and compassionate relationship between physicians, as well as all other members of the healthcare team, and their patients." It reflects attitudes and behaviors that are sensitive to the values in the cultural and ethnic backgrounds of others. The humanistic healthcare professional demonstrates the following attributes as summarized by the acronym IEC-ARES (as found on the Foundation's website):

Integrity – the congruence between expressed values and behavior
Excellence and clinical expertise
Compassion – the awareness, acknowledgment of the suffering of another
Altruism – the capacity to put the needs and interests of another before your own

Respect – the regard for the autonomy and values of another person
Empathy – the ability to place oneself in another situation, i.e., doctor
    as patient
Service – the sharing of one's time and resources with those in need,
    giving beyond what is required

Although the relationship with the patient has always been central to medicine, it may be the most neglected area of learning in residency training. Nowadays most residents estimate that they spend only 20% of their time actually interacting with patients. During training, personal discomfort, fatigue, time pressures, and team conflicts often erode this relationship to the point where residents become numb to the emotional needs of patients. This increased emotional buffering or distancing from patients and their suffering is the least adaptive and most damaging strategy used by residents to decrease personal levels of stress. It is a form of denial that precludes a unique possibility for supervised learning and for exploration of painful issues in care. Although technical medical care may be provided, no holistic healing takes place.

The growing emphasis on profit-driven, managed, and "high-tech" care may prevent residents from developing primary care, "real world" skills, from being exposed to a wide range of socioeconomic and health-related problems, and from providing continuity of care. One US study surveying practicing internal medicine graduates showed that only 42% were "fully satisfied" with their outpatient/primary-care training.[5]

Physicians who stop caring have low career satisfaction levels, more lawsuits, and difficulty establishing practices. What is more insidious and disturbing, when empathy disappears from work it also disappears from life at home with one's partner, children, and friends.

Some patients are indeed difficult, argumentative, demanding, or angry. Others are so ill or upsetting to our wish to cure that we avoid them. Some reawaken our conflicts with parents and siblings and leave us bewildered at our response. Others simply happen to be number 32 of 70 in a busy emergency shift. Yet residents who do not learn to maintain empathy in the face of such stress compromise their present and future ability to truly heal their patients.

Aim to learn as much as you can about patient and family-centered care, the key concepts for which are dignity and respect, information-sharing, participation, and collaboration. You can find an excellent resource at the Institute for Family-Centered Care (www.ipfcc.org).

GREEN DRESS

I wore my green dress because it was still a beautiful July and if she had opened the blinds, she too would have seen the sun outside. I was completely lost in the light blue of my office, reading in "Madness and Civilization" about the ship that sailed along the shore carrying all the "insane," when my pager went off. It was the first week of residency and C-L service was still quite slow.

I nervously pressed the hand-sanitizer on the wall outside her door so many times that a large amount of gooey liquid filled my palm and dripped on my shoes. The sharp smell made me sneeze and my hands were now so greasy that I almost dropped my black clipboard with pages of instructions about doing a psychiatric interview. I held it close to my chest like a holy book as I stepped into the room.

"You must be Jean! I'm from Psychiatry." I said enthusiastically, still rubbing my hands. The blinds were shut and it took my eyes a few seconds to adjust to the darkness. Jean was lying under the white sheets with her eyes closed. She did not move.

"Your team has asked us to see you. They have concerns about you refusing treatment and I'd like to ask you a few questions, if that's okay."

She opened one eye and inspected me up and down, but then looked away without a word. Her hair was purple and cut really short. I noticed a plastic bag on the chair that once held her belongings but now was torn, with her clothes falling out.

"I want to start by asking you about yourself," I continued, quite unsure about how to proceed.

Five minutes later, Jean was walking down the hallway in hospital booties dragging her IV-pole, with two nurses and me running after her. The second hospital gown she wore to cover the crack of the first one, flapped behind her like broken sails. She was swearing loudly at the walls but suddenly stopped and turned toward the nurses.

"And by the way," she shouted, pointing at me, "Tell Dr Wilson that I don't need to see the damn psychiatrist, especially not the green lady from the beach!"

And she steered toward the elevators.

SIGNS OF TROUBLE IN RELATIONSHIPS WITH PATIENTS

The following are signs of trouble in a resident's relationship with her patients:

- Lack of emotional response to tragedy; rote functioning without affect
- Increased anger toward patients manifested by rudeness, infantilization, and racist, sexist, ageist, or other disparaging or attempted humorous remarks
- Identification of patients by body part, disease, or room number
- Tendency to blame patients for illnesses or for physician-patient stalemates
- Rushed or perfunctory interviews; failure to obtain personal and social histories of patients
- Fantasies of a "problem patient" dying or moving away
- Increased authoritarian style or attempt to force treatment options or religious views on patients
- Denial of a patient's illness or pathological features despite evidence
- Emotional over-involvement or over-identification with patients (including sexual behavior; see guidelines regarding boundary violations)
- Avoidance behavior with certain patients
- Hiding behind the anonymity of rounds (i.e., not providing your name to the patient)
- Increased tendency to refer patients on, rather than deal with difficulties directly

Avoiding Boundary Violations[19]

The following guidelines suggest approaches for avoiding complaints of sexual misconduct and preventing boundary violations:

1 Avoid any behavior, gestures, or expressions that may be seductive or sexually demeaning to a patient.
2 Show sensitivity and respect for the patient's privacy and comfort at all times:

   • Do not watch a patient dress or undress.
   • Provide privacy and appropriate covers and gowns.
   • Knock before entering the room.

3 Obtain permission to do intimate examinations, offer explanations as to the necessity of the examination, and answer anticipated questions concerning the examination.
4 Use gloves when examining genitals.
5 Do not make sexualized comments about a patient's body or clothing.
6 Do not make sexualized or sexually demeaning comments to a patient.
7 Do not criticize a patient's sexual orientation.
8 Do not ask or make comments about potential sexual performance except where the examination or consultation is pertinent to the issue of sexual function or dysfunction.
9 Do not ask details of sexual history or sexual likes and dislikes unless related to the purpose of the consultation or examination.
10 Do not request a date with a patient. Do not text or email them.
11 Do not kiss a patient. Do offer appropriate supportive contact when warranted.
12 Do not engage in any contact that is sexual (from touching to intercourse).
13 Do not talk about your own sexual preferences, fantasies, problems, activities, or performance.
14 Learn to detect and deflect seductive patients and to control the therapeutic setting.

15 Maintain good records that document the necessity for intimate examinations or questions of a sexual nature as well as
the pertinent positive or negative clinical findings.

16 Patients have the right to have a third party present during
internal/intimate examinations if they wish, with the exception of life-threatening emergencies. Document the name of
this person. In some cases, the physician will be able to provide this third party. In cases where the physician is unable to
provide such a person, patients should be informed that they
may bring a person of their choosing with them. In nonemer-
gency situations, physicians have the right to insist that a third
party be present during internal/intimate examinations, and
to refuse to conduct this examination if the patient refuses
consent for a third party to be in the room.

17 Work on enhancing your skills when taking a sexual history.

For an excellent review, see P French, BASHH National guidelines –
Consultations requiring sexual history taking.[10]

Avoiding and Dealing with Doctor–Patient Communication Problems[11]

- Empathy can be nurtured as well as compromised. Recognize
  under what circumstances it might be absent in you (e.g., over-
  booked clinics), and try to change what you can.[12] A review article
  in *JAMA* tracked mood states, interpersonal reactivity, and empathy over the internship year and demonstrated a decline in trainee
  empathy over that period.[13] Don't let this happen to you.

- Recognize whether patients of a certain age or type repeatedly
  produce intense feelings in you (e.g., anger, sexual attraction, or
  sorrow), and try to determine whether they have hit a nerve in you
  ("countertransference") or whether they are projecting their feelings
  on to you to give you a taste of their negative experience.

- Pay more attention to the patient's experience and less to your own
  performance anxiety, which will diminish with clinical experience.

- Distinguish your or your patient's anger at the system from
  your anger with each other, so that it does not contaminate your

interaction. Agreeing with a patient's upset will make you an ally rather than an adversary and may defuse conflict. Don't take it personally!

- Keep a record or journal of your emotional responses to key residency developmental or "initiation" issues – for example, the first death of a patient (see below), first delivery, first bearing of bad news – and refer to it when you are feeling emotionally numb.
- Ask your program about onsite resources for enhancing interviewing and communication skills (coaching, workshops, electives).

DELIVERING BAD NEWS TO PATIENTS[20]

One of the most stressful aspects of clinical care is revealing a bad prognosis to a patient. Here are some strategies for delivering bad news:

- Bad news is best delivered when you have time for the patient. Make sure that you and the patient are reasonably comfortable; sit down. A pleasant room and private setting are extremely helpful.
- Watch patients for all-important nonverbal cues as to how they are listening to you. Be prepared for strong emotions and acknowledge them.
- Straightforwardness and lack of prevarication are essential. Be clear, honest.
- Keep medical terms to a minimum.
- Give patients the chance to be prepared for what you say: give them a warning that you are about to tell them something very difficult.
- Patients must be given time to express their fears and worries. Offer any hope that is realistic. They will need to understand the news in their own terms and realize how it is likely to affect their future.
- Be well prepared for the session: try to have a plan for disclosure before the interview, be as informed as possible about the

patient's problem, and know how to get answers for the patient if you cannot answer her questions. Know what the patient needs to do next.

- Be available and schedule a follow-up session even if you are about to refer the patient to a specialist. Patients will appreciate your ongoing concern.
- Do not be surprised if you are more worked up about the news than the patient is. Patients can show true resilience or complete denial in the face of seemingly disastrous news.
- Don't take calls, texts, or pages during this discussion.

THE WALL

Patient after patient, note after note. Patients were shuttled in and out of the clinic rooms in 15-minute intervals. My brain had become lulled into a monotony of patients with knee and hip pain. I filled out templated notes on each patient. When did the pain begin? How would you rate your pain on a scale of one to 10?

The next patient was new to the clinic. I introduced myself and proceeded with my objective questions, thinking more of my notes and the next patients I had to see than of the person in front of me. Ms. Z was 58 years old. She had severe end-stage osteoarthritis in her knees with remarkable deformities. I inquired about what she had tried for her knee pain. "No one ever told me to try physical therapy!" I took a step back and tried to explain the usual sequence of therapies that are recommended prior to having surgery. Within moments, she burst into tears. And my attitude of monotonous ambivalence disintegrated. I sat forward and placed a hand on her knee.

She explained that she lives alone and has no social support. Her knee pain has been unbearable, and she fears that she may not be able to support herself financially any longer. It took a split second of vulnerability to break down my wall, the wall that serves to protect my heart from the daily emotional stress of being a physician. This was the reminder that I desperately needed midway through my intern year: the crucial reminder of why I went into medicine.

OTHER TIPS TO ENHANCE COMMUNICATION WITH YOUR PATIENTS

- Do not expect the same level of stoicism from patients that you expect from yourself. Learn to recognize cultural and personality and more traditional sex-related differences in the expression of pain, anger, and grief.
- Make a point of chatting with your patients and try to learn at least one fact about their lives that will make them more human to you (e.g., the man with dementia on 8D used to be a composer).
- Let positive countertransference happen consciously and selectively (e.g., "That old lady in the emergency department hallway could be my grandmother ").
- Remember your own experiences of illness, loss, discomfort, and vulnerability. These may differ from those of your patients, but the memory will help to link you in understanding.
- Do not be afraid to let your patients express their emotions. If you are afraid, find out why in therapy, in supervision, or in a resident support or Balint-style group rather than refer the patients for psychiatric treatment. When appropriate, consider acknowledging your feelings to your patient (e.g., "I am tired today because I was on duty all night").
- Get to know your patient's family when possible, and try to be available for brief education sessions. This may help your patient cooperate with your treatment, which will diminish your workload.
- Identify your patients' psychosocial needs. After you have done the groundwork, you may want to recruit help from the departments of psychology or psychiatry, social work, or chaplaincy. But do not call them in simply because you do not want to deal with these needs. You must not dilute your responsibility to your patients.

- Study your referral patterns to see whether you avoid certain problems with patients.
- Keep informed about key psychosocial issues, which often manifest themselves in patients if you take the trouble to ask.
- Be sensitive to the patient's feelings of being undressed or exposed.
- Knock before entering a room.
- Maintain good eye contact with the patient; avoid taking excessive notes.
- Ask how the patient would like to be addressed (first name/title), and make sure he or she knows *your* name.
- Try to sit or stand at the same level as the patient so as not to be intimidating.
- If you have an accent, speak slowly.
- Increase cross-cultural awareness by asking about your patient's background, learning of new language skills, and reading. Where appropriate, use a professional translator or, if necessary, a family member.
- Don't get angry about noncompliance with medication or treatment.
- Explore the patient's fears, misconceptions, side-effects, and financial worries (re drug cost) instead.
- All non-compliance has a differential diagnosis just like the illness you're treating!
- Use open-ended questions, and don't interrupt.
- Ask the patient about fantasies ("What do *you* think it is?"), feelings, fears, and expectations about the illness. Find out what has changed in their functioning and what their expectations of you are.
- Make your explanations short, clear, and concise. Don't use jargon. Provide printed material if available.
- *Negotiate*, rather than dictate, management and the treatment plan with the patient, as an authoritarian stance may lower compliance.
- Offer the patient and her family self-help-group information for added support. See www.selfhelpgroups.org.
- Try to follow your patients right through their illnesses. You'll learn much more through offering continuity of care in both the inpatient and outpatient settings.
- Be open to a patient's wish to explore alternative forms of healing (like acupuncture or herbal medicine) as an adjunct to conventional

care, if it enhances his/her sense of control and self-care. Check out the National Center for Complementary and Alternative Health website, https://nccih.nih.gov/health/whatiscam.
- Ensure privacy.
- See the following website for additional resources in communicating with patients: Cambridge Guide to the Medical Interview: http://www.gp-training.net/training/communication_skills/calgary/guide.htm

A Word on the Use of Social Media in Patient Care – Proceed with Caution

The WMA (World Medical Association) urges its members to establish guidelines for their physicians addressing the following issues:

1 Maintain appropriate boundaries in the patient–physician relationship in accordance with professional ethical guidelines just as one would in any other context.
2 Study carefully and understand the privacy provisions of social networking sites, bearing in mind their limitations.
3 Physicians should routinely monitor their own Internet presence to ensure that the personal and professional information on their own sites and, to the extent possible, content posted about them by others is accurate and appropriate.
4 Consider the intended audience and assess whether it is technically feasible to restrict access to the content to predefined individuals or groups.
5 Adopt a conservative approach when disclosing personal information as patients can access the profile. The professional boundaries that should exist between the physician and the patient can thereby be blurred. Physicians should acknowledge the potential associated risks of social media and accept them, and carefully select the recipients and privacy settings.
6 Provide factual and concise information, declare any conflicts of interest, and adopt a sober tone when discussing professional matters.
7 Ensure that no identifiable information about your patient is posted in any social media. Breaching confidentiality undermines

the public's trust in the medical profession, impairing one's ability to treat patients effectively.

8 Draw the attention of medical students and physicians to the fact that online posting may contribute also to the public's perception of the profession.

9 Consider the inclusion of educational programs with relevant case studies and appropriate guidelines in medical curricula and continuing medical education.

10 Bring your concerns to a colleague when observing his or her clearly inappropriate behavior. If the behavior significantly violates professional norms and the individual does not take appropriate action to resolve the situation, physicians should report the conduct to appropriate authorities.

(See chapter 12 for a fuller discussion of guidelines for the use of social media.)

Advocacy and Social Justice

When considering humanistic and patient-centered healthcare more deeply, the concept of social justice should be kept at the forefront in terms of individual care, but also as linked to the care of vulnerable, stigmatized, or under-served populations in the context of public health. Social justice is based on the concepts of human rights and equity. Under social justice, all groups and individuals are entitled equally to important rights, such as health protection and minimal standards of income. The goal of public health is to minimize preventable death and disability for all.

Our contemporary understanding of social justice has been impacted by the 1948 United Nations Universal Declaration of Human Rights, which underscores the conditions needed for social justice. These include equal liberties and opportunities, a fair distribution of resources, and support for people's dignity and self-respect.

Residents are invited to review the social determinants of health to examine inequities in access to healthcare. Examples: Ask yourself, How does socioeconomic status affect my patient's treatment options and treatment adherence? How does my institution address the issues of marginalized people? Where in my training am I exposed to education around social justice and the social determinants of health? How is accessibility to care contingent on a person's civil rights? How are specific health interventions realigned in specific populations, and what might their differential effects be? How are healthcare resources allocated and payment of new treatments determined? How can communication strategies be improved to reach populations that have been historically stigmatized, oppressed, or marginalized?

One of the pioneers in working on issues of public health and social justice in medical education is Dr Martin Donohoe. His *Public Health and Social Justice Reader* is excerpted on the Public Health and Social Justice website (http://phsj.org). This site also contains terrific links to full curricula, publications, resources, and DVDs, which can be used for group discussion.

Getting the Real Story from Your Patient

The concept of narrative medicine suggests that patients will tell us their story, their way, if we are willing to receive it. There are ways to improve your narrative competence.[14,15]

PRACTICAL STRATEGIES FOR PRACTICING A MORE NARRATIVE-BASED MEDICINE

Family physicians have become intrigued with what Rita Charon has called Narrative Medicine and what her colleagues in the United Kingdom have called Narrative-Based Primary Care. My own experience in offering narrative workshops to primary-care physicians (or better yet, family physicians), is that they agree with the principles, but wonder how they can realistically incorporate strategies into a busy office "without opening up a whole can of worms." There are ways to improve your narrative competence – that is, your capacity to receive, interpret, co-construct, and bear witness to the stories your patients bring you. Here are some simple, practical strategies to try and then integrate into your doctoring style.

1   Charon starts her first patient visits with, "What would you like me to know about you?" before jumping into questions about symptoms. Try asking a more open-ended question like

this in a new assessment. You can allow a few minutes for the patient to present their concerns and still move into a more systematic, structured inquiry after that. If you need to contain the story, you can employ your usual time-management strategies, but make a point of telling the patient that you want to pick up the thread next time. Ask, "Have I missed anything?" at the end.

2 The average doctor interrupts a patient within 15 seconds. Make a point of letting the patient finish her thought before launching into the next question or comment.

3 Consider asking your patient to write a one-page "Impact of My Illness" document, which you will read and discuss with them and keep in the chart. This may be the first time your patient was ever asked how the illness has changed/interrupted the story they had imagined for themselves.

4 Add a final "S" to your SOAP (Subjective Objective Assessment Plan) notes – for Suffering. You don't have to write this down, but ask yourself if you have allowed room for the patient to talk about their distress or real concerns in each visit.

5 Find out one thing you didn't know about your patient's story in every visit. Who are they when they aren't ill? What are their interests, hobbies, the names of their grandchildren? Did you know that man with Alzheimer's used to be a composer?

6 Look for a metaphor or key word that emerges in your meetings that is unique to your working alliance. It may be found through a humorous exchange, but can become a symbol of the story you are constructing together over time.

7 View non-compliance as a blocked narrative, not as patient stubbornness. Get the real story. Non-compliance has a differential diagnosis like every other problem in medicine. You are definitely a character in that plot. Spending the time now will save both of you time later.

8 The next time you are troubled by a patient encounter, take 3 minutes to write down what happened. Write it the way you would tell a colleague, as a story with a beginning, middle, and end. Having it down on the page will allow you

the distance to see how your own story (expectations, time pressures, unresolved grief) has collided with your patient's. Most people are surprised how much story emerges in only 3 minutes and how it can facilitate personal reflection.

9   In a time of high-tech record-keeping, make a point of maintaining eye contact and not typing while the patient is speaking. Your body language conveys (or annuls) your receptiveness to a story. Think of other barriers to storytelling in your office (e.g., where or how chairs are placed, your answering non-urgent calls during appointments, etc. Change what you can!

10   The next time you feel bored with a patient, think about the question you haven't asked. Ask yourself what your unexamined assumptions about the patient are and revisit the moment in your shared story where the assumption took hold.

11   Regarding assumptions, give yourself a writing prompt: "People with tattoos are ..."; "Obese people are ..."; "Single mothers are ..." Stereotypes are really the unexamined stories we tell ourselves without realizing it.

12   When you're not sure what is going on with a patient, ask them, "What do you think is going on?" This is the story he is telling himself over and over about his symptoms. It may or may not give you a clue about etiology, but at the very least it will enlighten you as to his fears/worst-case plot scenarios.

13   Patients tell stories differently to doctors than they do to anyone else. Ask them, "How would others describe you?" If what they tell you doesn't match what you're seeing in your visits, then you've missed something important in their story.

14   From time to time, ask your patient, "What's the one thing you haven't asked/told me?" Chances are that's the story that matters most.

15   Before you see your next patient, take a moment with their chart. Take a deep breath. Ask yourself, "Where did we leave the thread of our story the last time?"

A symptom is not a story. A lab result is not a story. They may be the punctuation, but there's always more.

What about My Patient's Mental Health?[16]

One of the real downsides of hospital-based training, endless rotations, and a lack of exposure to continuity of care is that residents come to see their patients' suffering or onset of mental distress as "somebody else's problem" (Many order a "psych consult" if the patient even appears troubled or upset).

More commonly, residents and fellows learn to refer out if a patient has any psychiatric illness history at all. Psychiatric illnesses are sometimes seen as "not real illnesses," or not worthy of having time spent on them, or as "encumbrances" which complicate "real" medical care. This suggests a split between mind, brain, and body, which is clearly archaic, and will prevent you from becoming a holistic, humanistic physician who can help your patients over time, no matter what challenges emerge.

US statistics suggest that 18.6% of all US adults have a mental, behavioral, or emotional disorder (excluding developmental and substance-abuse disorders). Among US adults, 4.1% have a mental illness that results in serious functional impairment. One in five children either currently or at some point during their life has had a seriously debilitating mental disorder. (Source: National Institute of Mental Health, www.nimh.nih.gov.)

The link between physical and mental health is becoming increasingly clear. Patients who have had an MI accompanied by depression have an increased mortality risk of 3 to 17%. A cancer patient with untreated depression have an increased mortality risk of 39%. Individuals who are schizophrenic have a 50% greater risk of dying from cancer. A young individual with depression has a 20% greater risk of type II Diabetes.

The idea that a hospital or outpatient practice can separate out mental illness from ongoing medical care is unrealistic and misguided.

We need to identify mental illness early, prevent it where possible, destigmatize it, provide resources, and optimize the care of *all* of our patients. Teamwork is key and a flexible/accessible model of shared, collaborative care of mental health between doctors and mental health specialists works best for most physicians and their patients. Remember, all therapeutic (and collegial) relationships are built over time.

In June 2014, the Royal College of Physicians and Surgeons of Canada published a document called "Mental Health Core Competence for Physicians."[17] The principles and competencies of mental health are summarized in table 6.4 (used with permission), and are linked to each

Table 6.4 Mental Health Competencies[17,18]

Role	Principles	Competencies
Medical Expert	Physicians have a responsibility to provide comprehensive care, including mental wellness, to their patients. This includes understanding the mental health condition of their patients; to treat these conditions within their competence level; and to refer appropriately. Physicians practice a "shared decision making model" with patients and other supports (i.e., families) that the patient identifies as active partners Consideration of, and respect for, diversity and cultural safety are embedded in daily practice and care planning/programs. Care and recovery builds on the strengths, capacities and reality of each patient.	Physicians will have working knowledge of the symptoms, etiology, and basic treatment of mental health and addiction conditions that may influence a physical condition that they are treating. Physicians will detect/ recognize physical health conditions in patients who present with what appear to be mental health conditions. Physicians will recognize the signs and symptoms of basic mental health conditions most common to their specialty practice, i.e., • Anxiety disorders • Mood disorders • Psychosis • Addictions • Grief • Situational stress • Cognitive impairment • Sleep disorders Physicians will undertake mental health screening where applicable.
Communicator	Clear, honest and respectful dialogue about mental health matters is a mutual responsibility between physicians and their patients. All colleagues and patients with mental conditions are treated with respect. Mental health promotion is emphasized in patient encounters.	Physicians communicate with their patients with respect and without stigma irrespective of their mental health condition.
Collaborator	The physician trusts, values and seeks out the contribution of other relevant health professionals; they collaborate and learn	Recognizes and respects the diversity of roles, responsibilities and competencies of other professionals in relation

Table 6.4 (Continued)

Role	Principles	Competencies
	with other professionals to achieve better patient outcomes; they consider patients as an active partner.	to their own as it relates to mental health and addictions. Works with and learns from others to assess, plan, provide and integrate mental health and addiction care for individual patients or groups of patients (shared, integrated care).
Health Advocate	Promotes holistic health and encourages active participation of patients and other healthcare professionals as "agents of change for mental health."	Identifies opportunities for advocacy, health promotion and disease prevention to optimize the care of their patients with mental health conditions.
Scholar	The recognition and treatment of mental health conditions should be promoted throughout the medical education continuum and in research.	Identifies and integrates information and evidence related to the care of patients with mental health conditions in their specialty.
Professional	Physicians are aware of their own cultural attitudes and biases toward people with mental health conditions, and how these may impact patient care.	Recognizes through self-reflection the impact of their behaviors, attitudes and knowledge gaps that may negatively impact the quality of care and health outcomes of their patients with mental health conditions.

of the CanMeds physician roles of medical expert, communicator, collaborator, manger/leader, health advocate, scholar, and professional. The goal is to diagnose and treat mental health disorders with empathy, clinic rigor, and in a timely fashion.

Patient Safety

The old Latin saying "primum non nocere" means "first do no harm." Although all doctors want to be helpful to their patients, error and miscommunication result in patient injury and death every year. Researchers from the Rand Corporation, Stanford, UCSF, Johns Hopkins, the

ECRI Institute, and 21 international stakeholders examined the existing literature on clinical error and patient safety, and published their findings in 2013. They were able to recommend the effectiveness of patient safety strategies and to identify contexts and elements, which can inform rigorous discussion about patient safety.

For more information on quality improvement, go to www.rand.org for a summary of their recommendations, and search for "patient safety."

REMAINING SENSITIVE AND COMPASSIONATE ABOUT DEATH

Residents frequently report that, although they are often called on to confirm the death of a patient, they receive no guidelines on how to do so from a compassionate as well as a medicolegal point of view. It makes sense to request seminars on death and dying, as they have been shown to increase levels of confidence and empathy in residents caring for the dying.[13] (Check out www.epec.net for a continuing medical education program called Education for Physicians on End of Life Care by Linda Emanuel, MD. Many useful links are also provided.) In Canada legislation to allow physician-assisted suicide is underway. Visit www.cma.ca for ongoing, debates, dialogues, updates, guidelines, and support.

Death is confirmed by

- Dilated, fixed pupils
- No carotid pulse
- No heart sounds and breath sounds for over one minute.

When you have confirmed a death:

1 Take a quiet moment to acknowledge this patient's life and passage. Remember that it is an honor to be involved at the time of death of a human being, not a nuisance.
2 If family members are present, express your condolences in an unrushed fashion. (During your training, learn all you can about culturally different interpretations of death, burial, and mourning, so that you can be sensitive with patients' families around the death of their loved ones).

3 If the family is not present, speak to ward nurses who knew the patient about the best way to contact the patient's family. If appropriate, notify the staff physician supervising care, who may wish to make the call. If you call the family, identify yourself and ask for the next of kin. State at what time the patient died and whether you were directly involved in her care. Ask if the person would like to come in to be with the body, and notify the nurses of that decision. Reassure the family member that the individual died peacefully, with good nursing care.

4 Record in the patient's chart the date and time you were called and the above clinical data regarding confirmation of death.

Sample Charting

Called to pronounce death of Mrs X. Patient was unresponsive to verbal/ tactile stimulus. Pupils were fixed/dilated. No breath/heart sounds heard.

No carotid pulse felt. Patient pronounced dead at 23:42, 6 Nov. 2003.

5 Fill out the death certificate as soon as possible. Find out local regulations regarding signing the death certificate, for example, to distinguish coroner versus non-coroner cases. Speak to your chief resident or attending physician if in doubt.

6 If a clinical autopsy or postmortem is medically indicated, clarify the reasons with your attending staff or treatment team and seek written permission in a sensitive fashion from the next of kin or executor of the estate. Explain to the next of kin that an autopsy may prove useful in better understanding the patient's disease, but that family wishes will be respected.

7 If the death has shaken or upset you, be sure to talk to a trusted colleague in order to gain support. Do the same for them. Model for students and junior residents that death can be talked about. You may also want to write in your journal or do a piece of reflective writing on what happened.

TIP: *"As a senior resident, I find it invaluable to do a briefing with the trainees involved after every single death, expected or not."*

I Remember, by David Kopacz
(dedicated to Samuel Shem)

I remember Carl CD4=0 ring-enhancing lesions on his MRI
seizing the moment, in a bad way,
this stick of a man
teetered on the brink of death
then stepped back into life
he told me how he was going to buy some weights
get his strength back
buy some new clothes
then he asked me if I would come to his funeral when he died
overworked, scared, and guilty,
I said, "Yes."
I'm sure he's been dead for years
I remember the old black guy who had to urinate
he had cancer all over his body
because of his penile prosthesis the nurse wouldn't start the foley
twice during the night
I catheterized him he was crying quietly
saying "I have to go, I have to go."
4:37 a.m.
the beeper woke me
shoes still on, the nurse said I should hurry
he lay there dead
now, I mean now, while I am writing this, years later, now, I realize what he
    meant when
he said, "I have to go."
pronouncing him dead:
there is nothing like the hollow silence of the chest of the dead, "yes, this
    man is
dead" then, telling the family them crying me feeling out of place and
awkward
I remember Larry, 40 y.o. stroked-out alcoholic always pulling out the NG tube
and hissing the only word I ever heard him utter,
"Bitch!"
I remember the young gay man, dying AIDS and his partner
Smashing Pumpkins playing "Space boy" on

their tape player

now that song always reminds me of death

I remember the latino, X-IVDA, current AIDS and his infected wife

reverse isolation

I remember Maitreya's black man with AIDS and CMV retinitis

I was never sure if he knew I was there

that he was in a hospital

that he was dying in the hospital while I was there

his eyes roamed, disconjugate

the first FHV+ blood I drew

I remember the fifty-year-old stroked-out black woman whose blood I mingled with my own

through a needle stick

perhaps that is the source of my affliction ...

I remember the Middle-Eastern man with kidney failure and granules of white on

his chest

all I could think of was "uremic frost"

Dr. Troyer leans over

tastes his fingers,

"sugar!" he says

and I see the spilled sugar on his tray

he took a long time to die

I remember the young Latino alcoholic man with foam coming out of his mouth

like a champagne bottle

he died quickly

I remember long days and longer nights I remember rage, sadness, and a helpless feeling

of being trapped I remember a dream about smashing a patient's head into the pavement

I remember a patient in the VA ER tears running down his face without any sign

of emotion

I admitted him to the psych ward

that was definitely not normal

I remember the patient who I was convinced would hit me

it seemed inevitable,

I was the doctor ...
he was mad
I was the doctor
and I didn't know any better
I often remember saying to myself,
"I don't know any better."
I remember being at home for Christmas eating cereal tears running down my
face without any sign of emotion
that was definitely not normal

REFERENCES

1 Jellinek MS. Recognition and management of discord within house-staff teams. *JAMA*. 1986;256(6):754–5. http://dx.doi.org/10.1001/jama.1986.03380060080030.
2 Goldman L, Lee T, Rudd P. Ten commandments for effective consultation. *Arch Intern Med*. 1983;143(9):1753–5. http://dx.doi.org/10.1001/archinte.1983.00350090131022.
3 Tokarz JP, Bremer W, Peter K. *Beyond Survival: A Book Prepared by and for Resident Physicians to Meet the Challenge of the Impaired Physician and to Promote Well-Being through Medical Education*. Chicago: AMA Press; 1979.
4 Winter RO, Birnberg B. Working with impaired residents: Trials, tribulations, and successes. *Fam Med*. 2002;34:190–6.
5 Edwards JC, Marier RL. *Clinical Teaching for Medical Residents: Roles, Techniques and Programs*. New York: Springer; 1988.
6 Morrison EH. Yesterday a learner, today a teacher too. *Pediatrics*. 2000;105:235–43.
7 Wigle RD, Eisenhauer EE. Queen's University. Reprinted with permission.
8 Patterson F, Knight A, Stewart F, et al. How best to assist struggling trainees? Developing an evidence-based framework to guide support interventions. *Educ Prim Care*. 2013;24(5):330–9. http://dx.doi.org/10.1080/14739879.2013.11494197.
9 CMPA (ed). Strengthening inter-professional communication. *CMPA Perspective*; March 2011:10–2.
10 Rougas S, Gentilesco B, Green E, et al. *Twelve tips for addressing medical student and resident physician lapses in professionalism*. Early Online Medical Teacher; 2015:1–7.
11 From *Members' Dialogue* (CPSO), Nov. 1993. Reprinted with permission.

12 French P. BASHH National guidelines – Consultations requiring
    sexual history taking. *Int J STD AIDS*. 2007;18(1):17–22. http://dx.doi.
    org/10.1258/095646207779949989.
13 Peterkin AD. Encouraging empathy. [*Med Post Suppl*] *Curr Ther*. (Seaforth)
    1989;(Sept):6, 8, 34.
14 Ptacek JT, Eberhardt T. Breaking bad news: A review of the literature.
    JAMA. 1996;276(6):496–502. http://dx.doi.org/10.1001/jama.1996.
    03540060072041.
15 Bagatell R, Meyer R, Herron S, et al. When children die: A seminar series
    for pediatric residents. *Pediatrics*. 2002;110(2):348–53. http://dx.doi.
    org/10.1542/peds.110.2.348.
16 Peterkin AD. Practical strategies for practising narrative-based medicine.
    Can Fam Physician. 2011;58(1):63–4.
17 Mental Health Competencies for Physicians. June 2014. http://www.
    royalcollege.ca/portal/page/portal/rc/common/documents/policy/
    mhcc_june2014_e.pdf
18 Peterkin AD. Using reflective writing with students: Ten tips. *CAME
    Newsletter*, May 2010:6,12.
19 Hickson G, Pichert JW, Webb LE, et al. A complementary approach to
    promoting professionalism: Identifying, measuring and addressing
    unprofessional behavior. *Acad Med*. 2007;82(11):1040–8. http://dx.doi.
    org/10.1097/ACM.0b013e31815761ee.
20 Bellini LM, Baime M, Shea JA. Variation of mood and empathy dur-
    ing internship. *JAMA*. 2002;287(23):3143–6. http://dx.doi.org/10.1001/
    jama.287.23.3143.

CHAPTER SEVEN

One Size Does Not Fit All: Unique Concerns

A reviewer for this new edition suggested that this chapter (or at least separating out specific trainee populations) was obsolete. I wish this were true. Gender issues, race, and religious beliefs can all have an impact on the learning experience of residents pursuing training in North America. Here are some key considerations.

WOMEN

Back in 1989, when the first edition of this book came out, 44% of Canadian medical school graduates were women, compared with 6% in 1959 and 33% in 1981.[1] In 1990, 30% of all medical residents in the United States were women; by the year 2010 it was predicted that over half of all US physicians will be women, although the AMA Women Physicians Health Survey put the figure at 29.4%.[1] In 2003 the number of women enrolled in medical school surpassed 50% in many provinces in Canada and had reached 52% by 2007.[2] These numbers continue to climb in Canada and in the United States.[3]

More female medical students of course mean more female residents moving forward into the next decade. In most countries, women tend to choose primary care fields for specialization: internal medicine, pediatrics, obstetrics, gynecology, family practice, and psychiatry. Several studies have shown that in residency women tend to work more hours, experience more stress, and report more personal, emotional, and relationship problems than do their male counterparts.[4] They still intentionally postpone pregnancy because of perceived threats to their careers, despite a marked drop in fertility rates after age 35.[5] Women have a higher debt load on graduating and tend to earn less money in medical practice than do men.

Women have also been shown to have similar academic but better communication skills, and to experience fewer lawsuits and higher levels of career satisfaction than men.[6] (Some of these findings may be attributable to the fact that women show more candor in surveys on residency stress or may be more open to seeking help.) It is, however, important to recognize some of the unique pressures that women face during their medical careers that men do not experience, or may experience to a lesser degree.

Medicine in North America has been and continues to be a male-dominated field to which women have been obliged to adapt. Women residents have few female role models among teachers and administrators in their chosen career, and still only sometimes find the satisfying mentoring that all developing physicians require. Women in medicine experience what has been called "role strain," in that they are expected to conform simultaneously to cultural stereotypes of the feminine "caregiver " who will humanize a harsh medical technology and of the competent, competitive physician. This can lead to struggles with assertion, authority, and designatory tasks, called "role incongruity," as many leadership qualities are designated as stereotypically male.[7] Their hectic schedules often wreak havoc with the expectations they and others have of their capacity to manage the responsibilities of housekeeping, parenting, and supporting family members.

In the hospital setting, women nurses sometimes compete with or are less tolerant of women physicians. Colleagues may expect them to carry a higher female or pediatric patient load, and patients may doubt their credibility or not address them as "doctor." Sexual harassment by colleagues and patients is also a more serious problem for women residents than for men. In a sample of 599 female doctors, 77% reported being sexually harassed by patients at least once since becoming physicians (see also "Abuse and Harassment" in chapter 1).

Pregnancy and issues related to the timing of starting a family pose logistical and personal dilemmas for couples. An Amercian Medical Association study found that one-half of women physicians who had children had had their first, and one-quarter had had their second, child during residency.[8] Despite these facts, some US schools and programs still do not have formal maternity leave policies. (One study showed that only 80% of US obstetrics-gynecology programs had maternity leaves and 69% paternity leaves – and they are in the business of delivering babies!)[9] In Canada maternity benefits are in all residents' contracts, although the length of leave may vary from program to program. However, a pregnant resident may still encounter subtle and not so subtle expressions of resentment from colleagues who believe they will have to carry her clinical load.

Trends among Women in Medicine[4,10]

- Within a decade of completing training, one-third of women physicians will take maternity leave, and 24% prolonged leave for other reasons. Most will have shorter work weeks than their male counterparts.[11]
- Two-thirds of practicing women physicians in the United States have children.[4]
- A recent University of Michigan study found that over their careers, women lose $350,000 due to a persistent gender wage gap (Source: www.cirvitals.org).
- For the most recent trends regarding women in medicine, visit the Women Physicians Congress at the AMA, http://www.ama-assn. org/ama/pub/about-ama/our-people/member-groups-sections/ women-physicians-section.page.

Suggestions for Women

- Apply to a residency program that has a significant or growing representation of women, particularly in leadership roles.
- Review contract issues on maternity leave and time-sharing options before applying.
- Make an effort to form links with women colleagues. If you encounter an attending physician or lecturer who appears to have managed juggling family and career life successfully, ask to keep in touch with her from time to time. Find a mentor.

- Consider forming a women's residency support group or lecture series. Nominate a person in your hospital as a contact person for women's issues or grievances. Include medical students.
- PAR-BC has an excellent policy paper on pregnancy during residency (www.par-bc.org).
- Check out the Office of Women's Programs at AAMC.
- Investigate the services provided by national and international medical women's groups. Here are some useful resources for assisting the process:

  - American Medical Women's Association, Harassment and Gender Discrimination Resource and Information Service (www.amwa-doc.org and http://www.amwa-doc.org/our-work/initiatives/gender-equity-task-force/mission-and-position/)
  - Association of American Medical Colleges (AAMC), Women in Medicine homepage (www.aamc.org/members/wim/start.htm)
  - Canadian Women's Health Network (www.cwhn.ca)
  - www.MomMD.com
  - AMSA (www.amsa.org) Gender and Sexuality Committee (http://www.amsa.org/AMSA/Homepage/About/Committees/GenderandSexuality.aspx)

Pregnancy[12]

- Where possible, plan carefully the timing of your pregnancy. Notify your residency program director of your dates (preferably after 13 weeks) so that together you can plan a reasonable schedule (e.g., lighter rotations before delivery, outpatient rotations upon return).
- Stay safe – watch out for radiation/chemotherapy exposure.
- Take good care of yourself. Carry snacks. Ask for help if you're tired.
- Be open with colleagues about dates and continuing difficulties. Do not become apologetic or overcompensating.

- Maintain close ties with your obstetrician, general practitioner, or midwife in case you experience complications or need letters for sick leave or scheduling recommendations.
- Three months has been shown to be the minimum period that should be allotted for maternity leave to allow for adequate rest and reorganization and to take account of day care regulations on the age at which infants are accepted. The CIR (www.cirseiu.org) has prepared a highly recommended resource packet of union ideas, proposals, and programs called *Pregnancy in Residency: A Union Perspective*. Plan carefully, and well in advance, the support you need with the logistics around your delivery and child care. Consult your own housestaff or postgraduate medical office for guidance. The websites listed above also cover issues relevant to pregnancy and parenting (see, too, the section on parenting in chapter 5 for further suggestions).

INTERNATIONAL MEDICAL GRADUATES[12]

Historically, it has been difficult for internationally trained physicians to obtain their license or to find residency positions in North America. Once accepted into residency, international medical graduates (IMGs) face unique pressures. These issues are addressed in detail by the Educational Commission for Foreign Medical Graduates (www.ecfmg.org).

Not only do IMGs have to cope with the rigors of residency scheduling and high levels of responsibility, but they must also adjust to the medical hierarchy, to changed legal status as immigrants or refugees, and to a new country, culture, language, and ethical or religious system. Rules governing male–female dynamics may differ. Dress and personal hygiene codes may be more stringent or more relaxed. IMGs tend to be older and already have families. Family members may become isolated from the new culture and thus more dependent psychologically and financially on the resident, who thus becomes a caregiver at both home and work. Adjustment and adaptation to a new culture creates significant stress for anyone and results in culture shock.[13] The social isolation of foreign residents caused by the absence of family or their own sensitivity about cultural differences can put them at high risk.

Foreign-trained residents who have studied in centers equipped with less technology or fewer resources than those in North America may experience particular struggles over competence, whereas those who have come from settings similar to North American centers resent the assumption by some that they are less skilled. Many IMGs have been delayed – some for 10 years or more – in being accepted for internship because of restrictions related to language, medical qualifying exams, and citizenship requirements. Historically, some provinces and states have imposed restrictive contracts on IMGs that oblige them on completion of training to work for up to 4 years in an underserviced area. Increased remuneration for working peripherally may not compensate for the inconvenience to the physician and her family.

Many IMGs experience a marked status shift; the medical resident who is from a Third World country may become more wealthy and comfortable than ever before, whereas professors from some countries in Eastern Europe who must repeat all of their training to obtain accreditation are often devastated initially. Regional differences in patients' acceptance of visible minorities or of those who speak with an unfamiliar accent can be significant, and many IMGs experience hostile and racist reactions from the patients they are expected to treat.

North Americans who complete medical school abroad are not exempt from added strain during their residency. Although they return to a culture they have known, it has continued to evolve in their absence; indeed, they often return to a different medical system (e.g., the Mexican-trained resident who returns to American medicine). They may feel apologetic or inadequate for not having been accepted in a North American medical school or for having learned different or less technological protocols. Canadian-trained physicians who acquire residencies in the United States are often bewildered by non-universal medical care.

Suggestions for IMGs

- Apply to a residency program that has significant representation of, or a special entry program for, IMGs or refugees. Current physician shortages in Canada have led to an increased number of positions.

- Determine any contractual or practice-related restrictions before accepting an internship. If necessary, consult a lawyer, who can help you avoid being exploited.
- Form a support group with other IMGs to prepare for qualifying exams. For information on the ECFMG exams see www. ecfmg.org. You can also meet others in your situation at exam preparation courses.
- Find out about community resources for newcomers. The ECFMG also has IMG consultants you can speak with as part of their Acculturation Program.
- Seek a mentor who is also an IMG (perhaps someone from your own country or culture), or someone informed on IMG issues whom you can consult from time to time for advice and support.
- As you adapt to a new culture, maintain close social ties with your family and ethnic community. Attend organized events with your family.
- Keep your sense of humor!
- Anticipate religious and cultural holidays and ask for time off in advance.
- Find out about harassment policies at your school.
- Make friends with your North American colleagues – don't allow yourself to become ghettoized!
- Consider bringing a family member from your homeland for support or child care during your first year.
- Guard against a tendency to be overcritical of yourself because what you know is different. Ask questions and be open, rather than apologetic, about protocol differences. Ask your senior resident for intermittent one-on-one attention if you are weak in a particular area. Point out how you can enrich your program through your knowledge of other cultures and languages.
- Contact the national and international medical ethnic groups and associations. Your union may also have special committees and initiatives related to IMG training. (See other resources listed in chapter 13.)

- Online resources:

  - American College of Physicians – www.acponline.org (IMGs); http://www.acponline.org/about_acp/international/gradu-ates/practicing_in_us/programs.htm
  - American Council for Graduate Medical Education – www. acgme.org; http://www.acgme.org/acgmeweb/
  - American Medical Association – http://www.ama-assn.org/ ama/pub/about-ama/our-people/member-groups-sections/ international-medical-graduates.page
  - Educational Commission for Foreign Medical Graduates ECFMG) – www.ecfmg.org
  - Electronic Residency Application Support (for IMGs) – www. ecfmg.org/eras
  - Foundation for Advancement of International Medical Educa-tion (FAIMER) – www.faimer.org
  - International Federation of Medical Students (IFMSA) – http://ifmsa.org
  - Medical Graduates Educational Commission for Foreign Medical Graduates – www.ecfmg.org
  - www.mdspouses.com – An online community for spouses and families of IMGs
  - Canadian Information Centre for IMGs – http://www.cicic.ca/
  - Federation of Medical Regulatory Authorities of Canada (re licensing requirements) – http://www.fmrac.ca/
  - www.ethnicphysicians.org – Ethnic physicians organizations

VISIBLE MINORITY RESIDENTS

Special incentive programs for Aboriginal students in Canada and for black, Hispanic, and Native American students in the United States have produced a limited increase in their representation in the profession. These students sometimes encounter resentment in residency because frequently such programs are believed to constitute "reverse discrimi-nation or racism," that is, they are seen to give preferential treatment, or even exclusive access to medical training, to the participants solely because of their ethnic background. Many of these residents experience a socioeconomic and status shift, because they are more educated or better paid than many of their family members but are less affluent than or socioeconomically remote from their white resident counterparts. They may experience a unique kind of marginality that leaves them feeling suspect, or like "impostors," both at home and at work.

Residents whose skin color others perceive to be similar (e.g., those from a variety of Asian backgrounds) may be "lumped together " in the minds of patients and colleagues. As happens with IMGs, these residents may encounter subtle assumptions or biases in patients, colleagues, and support staff, sometimes in direct personal comments, sometimes in having patients from "their" presumed ethnic group referred to them.

RELIGIOUS RESIDENTS

Religiously observant or devout residents, whether Christian, Jewish, Muslim, Buddhist, Sikh, Hindu, followers of a Native traditional way, or others with strong spiritual convictions, may experience dilemmas about such matters as abortion, contraception, non-marital unions, and homosexuality when asked to carry out duties or confirm advice that they find immoral, unethical, or otherwise in conflict with their values.

Suggestions for Visible Minority and Religious Residents

* Apply to a residency program with significant visible-minority representation or a religious affiliation.
* Know your spiritual and cultural legacy and draw on it for strength. Talk to your spiritual leader/clergy about your life in residency.[14]
* Request religious holidays off well in advance and, if timely, explain the significance of the holiday to broaden your colleagues' worldviews.
* Consider finding a mentor with similar cultural or religious traditions so that you can share problem solving issues.
* Speak with the hospital ethicist or chaplain about the best way to make your views known to, and understood by, colleagues and patients.

- Challenge generalizations and stereotyping calmly when you encounter them clinically. You are in a unique position to educate ethnocentric or nonreligious physicians.
- Consider forming a support group with other residents whose background or tradition is similar to yours.
- Find "teaching moments" to talk about your cultural experience or religious tradition. You can actually help other residents to expand their worldview.
- Consider inviting speakers and holding seminars for the hospital at large on treating specific groups of patients. Offer to be a minority representative in your hospital.
- Although the system may encourage "tokenism," affirm your individuality and level of skill and resist the temptation to overcompensate or prove something.
- Contact resource groups for information on conferences, grants, minority research opportunities, and services.
- All residents should recognize that there is value in finding or rediscovering a spiritual or faith-related focus when facing the stresses and challenges of residency, as it can be an important source of sustenance and growth. Check out the following resources:

  - Robert Wood Johnson Foundation (www.rwjf.org)
  - Center for Spirituality and Health (www.spiritualityandhealth. ufl.edu)
  - George Washington Institute for Spirituality and Health (www. gwish.org)
  - Duke Center for Spirituality (www.spiritualityandhealth.duke. edu/)

Prayers on Healing

Here are some sample prayers on healing from different religious traditions.

The Prayer of Maimonides[15]

Almighty God! With infinite wisdom has thou shaped the body of man. Ten thousand times 10 thousand organs has thou put within it that move in harmony and without ceasing to keep in all its beauty the whole – the body, the envelope of the immortal soul …

To Man has thou given the wisdom to soothe his brother's suffering, to know his disorders, to extract what substances may heal, to learn their powers, and prepare and use them suitably for every ill … Inspire in me a love for my art and for thy creatures. Let no thirst for profit or seeking for renown or admiration take away from my calling … Keep within me strength of body and of soul, ever ready, with cheerfulness, to help and succor rich and poor, good and bad, enemy as well as friend. In the sufferer let me see only the human being … If those should wish to improve and instruct me who are wiser than I, let my soul gladly follow their guidance; for vast is the scope of our art …

In all things let me be content, in all but the great science of my calling. Let the thought never arise that I have attained to enough knowledge, but vouchsafe to me ever the strength, the leisure and the eagerness to add to what I know. For art is great, and the mind of man ever growing.

Almighty God! In thy mercy thou has chosen me to watch beside life and death in thy creatures. I now go to the work of my calling.

In its high duties sustain me, so that it may bring benefit to mankind, for nothing, not even the least can flourish without thy help.

Medicine and Illness[16]

Honor the doctor for his services, for the Lord created him.

His skill comes from the Most High, and he is rewarded by kings.

The doctor's knowledge gives him high standing and wins him the admiration of the great.

The Lord has created medicines from the earth, and a sensible man will not disparage them. Was it not a tree that sweetened water and so disclosed its properties?

The Lord has imparted knowledge to men, that by their use of his marvels he may win praise; by using them the doctor relieves pain and from them the pharmacist makes up his mixture.

There is no end to the works of the Lord, who spreads health over the whole world.

My son, if you have an illness, do not neglect it, but pray to the Lord, and he will heal you.

Renounce your faults, amend your ways, and cleanse your heart from all sin.

Bring a savoury offering and bring flour for a token and pour oil on the sacrifice; be as generous as you can.

Then call in the doctor, for the Lord created him; do not let him leave you, for you need him.

There may come a time when your recovery is in their hands; then they too will pray to the Lord to give them success in relieving pain and finding a cure to save their patient's life.

When a man has sinned against his Maker, let him put himself in the doctor's hands.

A Physician's Prayer

Dear Lord, give skill to my hand, clear vision to my mind, kindness and sympathy to my heart. Give me singleness of purpose, strength to lift at least a part of the burden of my suffering fellow mortals and a true realization of the privilege that is mine. Take from my heart all guile and worldliness that with the simple faith of a child I may rely on thee. Author Unknown

Maimonides' Code for Physicians[17]

O god, may the love of my art actuate me at all times; may neither avarice, nor miserliness, nor the thirst for glory or a great reputation engage my mind, for, enemies of truth and philanthropy, they could easily deceive me and make me forgetful of my lofty aim of doing good to thy children. Endow me with strength of heart and mind, so that both may be ready to serve the rich and the poor, the good and the wicked, friend and enemy, and that I may never see in the patient anything else but a fellow creature in pain.

If physicians more learned than I wish to counsel me, inspire me with confidence in and obedience toward the recognition of them, for the study of the science is great. It is not given to one alone to see all that others see. May I be moderate in everything except in the knowledge of this science; so far as it is concerned, may I be insatiable; grant me the strength and opportunity always to correct what I have acquired, always to extend its domain; for knowledge is boundless and the spirit of human kind can also extend infinitely, daily to enrich itself with new acquirements.

GAY AND LESBIAN RESIDENTS

Gay and lesbian residents, who make up an estimated 10% of the resident population, not only face particular challenges in their daily lives, but also must deal with a medical hierarchy that can at times be rigid and intolerant. Gay men and women historically have been an invisible, rejected minority, and those in most residency programs still find it necessary to hide their sexual identity from colleagues. This results in social isolation, stigmatization, and missed peer support about shared issues, such as couple relationships.

The gay resident's partner may experience increased isolation because of a reluctance on the resident's part to socialize with colleagues, which may produce added couple conflict. The gay resident lacks public role models who are comfortable with their own professional and sexual identities, and therefore may not find a mentor.

Gay residents can be victims of social or sexual harassment from superiors, but may remain silent to protect their own identities. They may let homophobic remarks by patients and colleagues go unchecked for fear of disclosing their orientation and thereby attracting hostility or suspicion. Such situations result in much unresolved anger.

Gay residents working with children in pediatrics or psychiatry may experience particular stress or feel suspect because of the common and unfounded misconceptions that homosexuals may "contaminate" or molest children. Those considering a career in psychiatry will often be asked about sexual orientation before they enter a residency and/or will be assumed to be heterosexual by the professors who supervise their psychotherapy.

Some residents report being refused entry to specific programs because of perceived homosexuality or HIV-positive status. The gay male resident in medicine or surgery may experience marked anxiety when treating patients with AIDS because of his own fear of the disease as a member of a hard-hit community or because he or his lover is HIV-seropositive. He may also be worried about meeting social contacts clinically or patients socially.

Finally, many men and women only start to come to grips with their gay identity during the years they spend in residency. Regrettably, training demands can delay such important discoveries and personal growth. The experience of transgender residents is as yet under-documented but needs to be a part of this discussion over time.

Suggestions for Gay and Lesbian Residents

- Contact the Gay and Lesbian Medical Association (www.glma. org) and the local gay press for notices of meetings of gay health-provider organizations in your city. These groups are welcoming to bisexual and transgendered members as well.
- Choose a residency program in a city with an active and political gay life. Such a city will also have a higher visible percentage of gay physicians who can help you in your career and serve as role models.
- As you get to know other residents and interns you will gradually perceive whom you can tell about your life. Do not shut yourself off from possible peer support for you and your partner.
- Do not feel obliged to let homophobic remarks go unchecked. Respond firmly and calmly. Use the situation as an opportunity to educate.
- Resist any tendency to overcompensate because of being gay or lesbian. If you are having particular difficulties with reconciling your sexual and professional identities, seek help in the form of psychotherapy.
- Remember that you are not obliged to answer questions pertaining to sexual orientation in residency applications or employment interviews. The choice is yours.
- Encourage your program to provide sensitive, appropriate training regarding the care of gay, lesbian, and transgendered patients. For further reference to these and related issues, see Peterkin and Risdon's *Caring for Lesbian and Gay People*.[18]

RESIDENTS WITH A DISABILITY, CHRONIC ILLNESS, OR LEARNING CHALLENGE

Residents who are blind, use wheelchairs, or have a chronic illness (such as diabetes, chronic pain, lupus, or asthma) experience increased stress as a result of their disability that may in turn be worsened by residency-related stress. Residents with a visible impairment may have to work harder to establish credibility with patients and to deal repeatedly with social awkwardness in patients and colleagues in a way that sometimes wears down a successful coping style. Colleagues, in particular, may try to be over-helpful or may be reluctant to acknowledge the disability. Precedents of residents with most disabilities (including blindness, quadriplegia, and learning difficulties) now exist, but program directors may still be worried about these residents' "efficacy and suitability" for the specialty.

The resident who becomes seriously ill during residency must contend with issues of loss, pain, and uncertainty, in addition to the stresses of residency.

Suggestions for Residents with a Disability, Chronic Illness, or Learning Challenge

- Good support from family, other housestaff, and hospital support staff is essential. Calculate the help you need regarding such matters as navigation, elevator service, and special meals, and request it. Never ask someone junior to you to make decisions for you. Try to form particular ties with porters, orderlies, nurses and nurses' aides, mail carriers, and elevator operators, who will probably be glad to help.
- Discuss your disability or illness openly with your program director and chief resident so that she can help you develop strategies. Do not hide periods of illness from colleagues, as such stoicism may compromise your own and your patients' care.
- Maintain close links with your personal physician so that you can get quick follow-up, treatment, and letters for sick leave or change of duties if required.

- Some patients are comforted to learn that their physician is not omnipotent and shares the experience of illness. Avoid the tendency to overcompensate, to neglect your personal life, or to be a "super-doctor" because of your disability, but remember that you may have something to teach your housestaff team about the experience of being a patient.
- Find out about program resources and accommodations for learning difficulties and how to access them.

For information on resources for disabled doctors:

- In the United States, go to the US. Equal Employment Opportunity Commission (www.eeoc.gov).
- In Canada, go to the Canadian Association of Physicians with Disabilities (www.capd.ca).

REFERENCES

1 Etzel SI, Egan RL, Shevrin MP. Graduate medical education in the United States. *JAMA.* 1989;262(8):1029–37. http://dx.doi.org/10.1001/jama.1989.03430080049007.
2 *Maclean's.* 24 Sep 2007:62.
3 http://www.acgme.org.
4 Bickel JA. Women physicians: Change agents or second-class citizens? *Humane Med.* 1990;6:101–5.
5 Willett LL, Wellons MF, Hartig JR, et al. Do women residents delay childbearing due to perceived career threats? *Acad Med.* 2010;85(4):640–6. http://dx.doi.org/10.1097/ACM.0b013e3181d2cb5b.
6 Borsellino M. Female MD time off the job creates uncertainty for manpower planners. *Med Post,* 27 Mar 1990.
7 Bartels CB, Goetz S, Ward E, et al. Internal medicine residents' perceived ability to direct patient care: Impact of gender and experience. *J Womens Health (Larchmt).* 2008;17(10):1615–21. http://dx.doi.org/10.1089/jwh.2008.0798.
8 Franco K. Conflicts associated with a physician's pregnancy. *Am J Psychiatry* 1983;140(7):902–4. http://dx.doi.org/10.1176/ajp.140.7.902.
9 Davis JL, Baillie S, Hodgson CS, et al. Maternity leave: Existing policies of obstetrics and gynecology residency programs. *Obstet Gynecol.* 2001;98(6):1093–8. http://dx.doi.org/10.1016/S0029-7844(01)01605-2.

10 Finch S. Pregnancy during residency. *Acad Med.* 2003;78(4):418–28. http://
    dx.doi.org/10.1097/00001888-200304000-00021.

11 Barzansky B. Educational programs in U.S. medical schools 2001–2002.
    JAMA. 2002;288(9):1067–72. http://dx.doi.org/10.1001/jama.288.9.1067.

12 Walsh A, Gold M, Jensen P, et al. Motherhood during residency training.
    Can Fam Physician. 2005;51:990–1.

13 Alguire PC, Whelan GP, Rajput V. *The International Medical Graduate's Guide
    to US Medicine & Residency Training.* Philadelphia: American College of
    Physicians; 2008.

14 Kaplan HD, Sadock BJ. *Comprehensive Textbook of Psychiatry.* 7th ed. Balti-
    more: Williams and Wilkins; 2005: 1412–13.

15 Etziony ME. *The Physician's Creed: An Anthology of Medical Prayers, Oaths
    and Codes of Ethics Written and Recited by Medical Practitioners through the
    Ages.* Springfield, IL: CC Thomas; 1973: 29–30.

16 *Jerusalem Bible,* Eccles. 38:1–15.

17 *The Code of Maimonides.* New Haven, CT: Yale University Press; 1949.

18 Peterkin AD, Risdon C. *Caring for lesbian and gay people: A clinical guide.*
    Toronto: University of Toronto Press; 2003.

CHAPTER EIGHT

Whiz Kids: Teaching, Learning, Doing Research, and Leading with No Time

LEARNING

Effective study seems virtually impossible when you are tired or overworked. Decreased sleep, anxiety, physical discomfort, and high noise and distraction levels have variable effects on the desire to learn, memory, reading capacity, concentration, and task performance. The housestaff member who has a weekend or evening off is unlikely to study because of a need for sleep or social contact; he or she may then feel guilty and inadequate. Try to study when you are relaxed, as you will learn and retain more. Medical information has never been easier or quicker to obtain online, so you can access it wherever you are, whenever you want![1]

TIP: "For internal medicine residents especially, it is important to keep up on developments in diagnosis and therapy. At the very least, it is important to keep track of journal articles via, e.g., email or RSS feeds if not actually read a journal regularly."

Be aware of your preferred learning styles and which one to use in different circumstances. (Most people's learning styles draw on one or two behaviors that they prefer to others.) Knowing this will help you to keep up learning throughout your medical career, and in selecting/accessing appropriate continuing medical education (CME) options.

Basic Learning Styles

- Using examples from concrete experience (e.g., in-class case studies)
- Observing, listening, and reflecting (e.g., after doing rounds)
- Working with abstract concepts, relying heavily on logic for analysis and theorizing (e.g., studying texts and debating with colleagues and teachers)
- Learning by doing, active experimenting, and practicing (e.g., making diagnoses, performing procedures, and working with patients)

CONTINUING MEDICAL EDUCATION

Definitions and Options[2,3]

The American Medical Association and the Accreditation Council for Graduate Medical Education (ACGME) define CME as follows: "Continuing medical education consists of educational activities that serve to maintain, develop, or increase the knowledge, skills, and professional performance and relationships that a physician uses to provide services for patients, the public, or the profession. The content of CME is that body of knowledge and skills generally recognized and accepted by the profession as within the basic medical sciences, the discipline of clinical medicine, and the provision of health care to the public" (AMA Policy Statement 300.988; http://www.ama-assn.org). The Royal College of Physicians and Surgeons of Canada now requires credits for maintenance of certification (see http://www.royalcollege.ca/portal/page/portal/rc/members/moc), as does the College of Family Physicians of Canada (http://www.cfpc.ca/mainpro/). Increasingly, continuing medical education will become a mandatory part of maintaining licensing in most jurisdictions.

Self-Directed CME Methods

- Reading journals, texts
- Computer (online) programs – often free through your university or watch for discount coupons!
- Clinical traineeships
- Teaching
- Publishing

- Literature searches
- Audio or videotapes
- Self-assessment and needs assessment programs
- Research
- Self-audit of practice

TIP: "It is important to beware of the bias inherent in sources and teachers. Residents should feel free to ask presenters for disclosures, and beware of 'incentives' (dinners, etc.) from industry. There is a large body of literature showing that these things make a difference in prescribing practice."

Group CME Methods

- Grand rounds
- Conferences
- Audits of practice
- Structured formal examinations
- Journal clubs
- Workshops
- Self-assessment programs
- Quality assurance programs

The Call Cycle, by Emily R. Transue

1. On Call
Sometimes the busy moments
Are the easy ones.
Not the crazy times
When your pager keeps exploding
And the admits pour in
And the chaos unconcentrates
And you hope to hell you won't kill somebody
By mistake, distraction, oversight but the quiet moments are bad, too;
Too much time to think
To wonder when the next one's coming in
Whether you'll sleep the night through
Or get three hits at three a.m.
Time to be afraid of what you should've done and didn't

What you did do and should not have
In the wakeful silence, head on pillow.
The best times were
Just working, steadily,
Doing what is needed but not
More than can be done;
Riding the momentum of necessity,
Busy, numb.

2. Morning After
Green moss
Pebbles
A bit of broken glass;
Further off, a patch of yellow lichen.
It is so wet
And so clear
I'd swear that I can smell it through the glass,
That other world
Outside this window
Where linger at the elevator dawdles.

After all these hours here
The smell of hospital is in my pores.
I wish the window opened.
I'd like to breathe the air.

3. Afternoon After
Have you ever been so tired
You could cry, just from fatigue?
So tired that voices hurt your ears
And you'd like to curl up in a little ball
Under a lake or a rock
And die
If dying means to sleep forever.

4. The Day Between
My family thinks
If you're not "on," you're "off."

It's hard to argue
Hard to explain

That a day of work
With sleep before and after
Is luxury enough.

5. Pre

This morning I rounded on
Two patients in my care a month each
On ventilators,
Patients who have never spoken to me.
A woman whose abdominal pathology
All of modern medicine has failed to diagnose,
Another whose lymphoma all of modern medicine has failed to cure,
A third who will recover from her cellulitis,
Go home, shoot up again, come in again.

I was screamed at by the brother of a man
Who's dying of hepatic carcinoma at 41;
He yelled at me because he couldn't yell at God

Then I went to clinic, to see
A woman with diabetes without a home
Who's struggling against despair
And a man who wanted prescriptions
And someone to laugh at his jokes
And an alcoholic who needs a detox bed
But won't get one
Because the city has none empty.

I leave the radio off, driving home,
Because I cannot stand to hear another voice, another noise.
I sit on my sofa, still,
My mind a blank;
I am
An eggshell
Or a melon rind:
Scooped out,
Round and empty.
I've given all I have; there's nothing left.
I soak in a hot bath and go to sleep.

Making the Most of Your Learning Potential

Identify your own preferred learning style, as described above. Try to read up on a subject before a lecture to enhance learning. During teaching rounds, concentrate on taking away one new fact from each seminar. Learn something new every day.

At the beginning of your residency, reading about the cases you are actually treating provides a natural motivation. Make a note of questions and knowledge gaps as you go. Carry useful pocket manuals or your smart phone/iPad/laptop so that concisely organized facts are readily accessible. Subscribe to one or two good peer-reviewed, indexed journals in your field (either hard copy or online) and read the review articles. Find out what your hospital and university libraries provide in terms of journals, online resources and links, search engines and search assistance, and downloads.

If a synopsis of your large specialty textbook is available, read it and answer any review questions it contains. Use the large textbook for a more thorough review of a topic.

When asked to prepare a grand rounds, pick a practical, non-esoteric topic that you want to learn about. Concentrate on evidence-based clinical articles. Ask to incorporate "mini rounds" into morning rounds (e.g., a 5-minute presentation on a useful topic every morning). Do not be afraid to ask questions during rounds; you are there to learn.

Insist on proper supervision by attending staff. Recently the Joint Commission of Accreditation of Healthcare Organizations and the ACGME beefed up resident supervision rules, making it mandatory that medical staff be aware of these changes.

Carry a notebook or smart phone/iPad to jot down questions and useful facts, pointers, tables, and normal laboratory values. Try to play a teaching role with juniors and medical students; this will force you to review and present data clearly.

TIP: *"I have found it helpful to focus as much as possible on learning, during residency, skills that will probably not change (physical exam, history taking, physiology) and maybe even short-changing learning information that will change (e.g., guidelines which I can look up, medication doses for uncommon medications)."*

Identify gaps in your learning and arrange activities to fill them. Senior residents and program directors will have useful suggestions and resources. For instance, push for rotations in primary care, "free" or public health clinics, community and health centers; otherwise your training may be incomplete for practice in a nonhospital setting (i.e., "the real world"). Arrange occasional individual teaching sessions with a mentor or tutor. You may have to request such sessions if your program does not offer them.

If your contract allows it, arrange to take time off every year for study, conferences, and exam preparation. Consider using this time to take a specialty review or exam preparation course.

Spend time developing an efficient Internet search strategy. Conduct regular searches on topics of interest. Two excellent resources are the ACP Journal Club (Evidence-Based Medicine for Patient Care – www. acpjc.org) and the Cochrane Collaboration – www.cochrane.org.

EXAMS!

One of the greatest stresses of residency involves preparing for, and then taking, the written and oral qualifying exams (the "boards") associated with internship, residency, or subspecialty fellowship. Since you're already preparing, you might wish to take qualifying exams in both Canada and the United States to keep all your options open.

Study and Exam Preparation Tips

- Find out what your program offers by way of mock oral exams, old exam questions, online study guides, and exam review courses.
- Find out application deadlines for written and oral exams. Don't miss the deadline! As the exam draws near, form a study group with three or four friends whose study styles are similar to yours.

- Consider every patient you see to be a potential case presentation for your exam. Discipline yourself to do a thorough history, physical, and case formulation about your patient. Practice presenting the case formally to a teammate from time to time.
- Remember to read about specific cases and actively protect study time throughout your residency.
- Emphasize problem solving rather than memorization, but remember to review rare disease entities and the basic medical sciences of your specialty (i.e., physiology, biochemistry), as you may be asked questions about these in the written and oral exams.
- Try to obtain past fellowship or board written exams and work through them alone or with your study group.
- Find out about board reviews offered by your program or intensive exam workshops offered at other national centers.
- Arrange mock oral exams with senior clinicians in your department at least once a year and request detailed written and verbal feedback.
- Talk to recent candidates about the content and format of their exam.
- To avoid "study burnout," reward yourself, for example, with an outing or special meal when you've had a productive session.
- For information on exam step 3 of the United States Medical Licensing Exam (USMLE), see www.usmle.org.
- In Canada, exam links are:
  - LMCC-2: http://mcc.ca/examinations/
  - Royal College of Physician and Surgeons: http://www.royalcollege.ca/portal/page/portal/rc/public; http://www.royalcollege.ca/portal/page/portal/rc/credentials/start
  - College of Family Physicians of Canada: http://www.cfpc.ca/ExamInformation/
- If you don't pass, be kind to yourself. You can take the exam again.

CHANGING POSITION

Being a left-handed surgery resident was more difficult than I had anticipated. But I was beginning to feel obtuse, awkward, and hesitant outside of the operating room as well. Figuratively and literally it was apparent that I was not fitting in.

A patient complication. A harsh senior resident. A failed exam. An argument with a friend after I went to him for help ("You've been so sensitive lately, and it's really annoying.") The physical exhaustion was eventually replaced by a mental and spiritual exhaustion. I didn't think I could continue.

The stresses of surgical residency are unique. For many, surgical residency represents our first experiences with personal failure. The fact that many of these failures are not preventable does little to appease our consciences. We are committed, high-achievers, and reconciling with our own shortcomings takes both effort and humility. We often work twice as long as our colleagues, and receive half the praise. Double standards for expectations can be pervasive, within our own department and throughout the rest of medical culture.

One day in the operating room, a staff member suggested to me: "Why don't you try standing on the opposite side of the table. I think it will be easier for you." He was right. The steps of the operation flowed better. I gained confidence. I took pride in my work, and my performance improved.

I began to reposition and refocus myself from a mental and spiritual perspective, as well. The senior resident was a new mother, with a 6-month-old infant at home. I studied for and repeated the exam with a friend who was also unsuccessful (we had been too ashamed and embarrassed to admit it to each other.) The other resident who admonished me had his own stresses, and once we discussed them, he became my gym buddy. I focused on small successes, instead of ruminating on my failures. I felt better equipped to continue my residency. Though work was still difficult and expectations remained high, I had reclaimed the joy that had been fostered years ago when I was a medical student.

Breathe. Take a few steps. Reposition yourself to approach a challenge from the opposite direction. You may be surprised what you discover.

Test Taking Tips

1 Get to know the material.
2 Get enough sleep.
3 Follow a normal routine the day of the exam.
4 Take deep breaths!
5 Wear comfortable clothing.
6 Arrive early enough to sign in and take the time allotted.
7 Check the test brochure to be certain that you bring all needed documents (e.g., admission card or identification with picture).
8 Be familiar with the test format (i.e., take a computerized practice test and the tutorial on the CD supplied with the registration materials).
9 Be familiar with the types of questions (short answer, multiple choice) that will be asked.
10 Know how the test will be marked.
11 Watch the clock.
12 Use your time efficiently.

(*Source*: Iserson KV, *Iserson's Getting into a Residency: A Guide for Medical Students*, 7th ed. Tucson, AZ: Galen Press; 2006.)

TEACHING

One of the enduring ironies in postgraduate medical education is that staff physicians teach residents and residents teach medical students, but it seems in most programs that nobody teaches anybody *how* to teach. As a result, the caliber of teaching residents receive varies significantly from school to school, hospital to hospital, and attending to attending.[4]

Teaching occurs at the bedside, on rounds, in conference rooms, in journal clubs, on grand rounds, and at conferences, but most residents are hard-pressed to describe their own learning style (see above), much less which attributes make for an effective teacher. Residents generally emulate "good teachers" and promise themselves not to be like "bad teachers." Many postgraduate medical offices provide workshops and tutorials on teaching, and some staff physicians make a point of teaching about teaching. One useful program offered at centers across Canada and the United States is the Teaching Improvement Project System (TIPS). Here following are practical suggestions for maximizing teaching and learning in a variety of settings.

TEACHING

One of my senior residents liked to give PowerPoint presentations. Several times a week, she would bring her tiny MacBook to the hospital. We crowded around a table and listened to her talk. Another senior resident liked to hand out papers. By the end of our month together, my knapsack had seemingly doubled in volume and weight from the papers he printed.

I remember hardly anything about what they taught, only how they taught it. I do remember their styles and their actions: the resident who made sure to learn every nurse's name, and the one who made us present our cases in front of our patients, letting the patients jump in when we made a mistake.

Also, I remember techniques I saw them apply: a senior resident who could focus so intensely on a patient the rest of the world seemed to vanish, or the neurology resident who showed me how, if you landmarked just right and took a moment to visualize the space, your lumbar punctures would hit home every time.

When I became a senior resident, these were the people I modeled myself upon. I tried to do the things I'd liked, and avoid the things I didn't. At least, I figured, I'd only make new mistakes. I try to be careful around my students. I know that they're watching my actions, ready to make them their own.

How to Maximize Bedside Teaching

It is surprising that less than 20% of resident time is actually spent at the bedside, but this time is vital for trainees to learn about patient interviewing, communication skills, and the art of the physical exam. Remember to:

- Model respect for the patient's privacy and wishes; keep visits brief.
- Introduce the patient to team members by name and give the names of your team members. Express gratitude for her time and assistance in teaching.
- Tell your team members in advance what you want them to observe or examine regarding the patient, so as not to linger at the bedside unnecessarily.
- Discuss the patient's case in a confidential fashion and setting (i.e., never in the elevator or cafeteria).
- Observe students' or juniors' physical-exam and interviewing skills wherever possible and provide immediate, one-on-one feedback.
- Your day is full of "teachable moments." Seize the moment!
- Schedule 5-minute "mini-rounds" on a useful topic during every morning round. Seize as many teaching opportunities as you can in the course of the day.
- Work to create a comfortable learning environment where ridicule, criticism, and unhealthy competition are not found. Be open to questions and feedback yourself.
- Provide suggestions for reading and learning more.
- Your specialty association website will likely have links on teaching.
- Go to https://www.mededportal.org (an AAMC initiative) for information and resources on teaching.

How to Give Verbal Feedback to a Trainee

- Make your expectations known for medical students, interns, and junior residents at the beginning of the rotation and refer to these throughout.

- Always focus your comments on specific performance observations, behaviors, or events rather than making subjective
  generalizations.
- Find an approximate time and quiet setting for discussion.
  Never humiliate publicly.
- Focus on what needs to be changed. Be succinct and direct and
  don't provide too much information.
- Frame your comments in an empathetic, constructive fashion,
  emphasizing patient care, teamwork, and common goals for the
  patient – avoid "put downs," blaming, or "ego challenges."
- Make your comments solution-based. Try to have the trainee
  elicit specific actions, decisions, or changes that would result in
  improved performance.
- Ask the trainees what they plan to do differently next time.
- Give frequent feedback and follow up on previous discussions.
- Familiarize yourself with your program's resident evaluation forms so you know what specific elements to look for in a
  trainee's performance.
- See also PARO's Top 10 Teaching Tips: http://www.myparo.
  ca/During_Residency#Teaching and find up-to-date references
  on teaching at http://residentteachers.usc.edu/

PROCEDURES

I have never been quick to learn procedures. Although I'm
an internal medicine resident, I couldn't consistently draw a
blood gas until the end of internship. The first joint aspirations
I did drew nothing but blood.

I eventually became comfortable with everything but central
lines. Something always went wrong and someone else always
had to take over.

This changed after I spent time on call in the ICU with Mark,
one of the fellows. The first time he saw me fail, he frowned,
scrubbed in, and slid the line in immediately.

"I'm sorry," I said.

"You need to stop being so tense," he said. "You just have to practice."

After scrubbing out, he opened a fresh kit and walked me through each step. When we reached a step where my hands failed, he made me repeat it until they didn't. This culminated in him watching me tie the knot which sutures the line in place.

"You do that, you'll stab yourself," he said. He took the suture and tied a perfect knot: slowly, so that I could see each step.

"Now, you do it," he said.

I fumbled my way through the tie, but got it.

He took the suture back from me and stuck the needle through my scrub top and another perfect knot.

"Now, do it a hundred times," he said.

Eventually, my lines began to go in smoothly, I became a senior resident, and began to teach interns. They fumble, the way I did; some more, some less. I always say the same thing.

"Relax," I say. "You just have to practice." Then I find the tools and we do it again.

Maximizing Conference Room Teaching

- Start and finish on time.
- Use audiovisual materials (including X-rays, scans, photographs) wherever possible to illustrate case material.
- Talk about people, not lab results. Keep the story interesting. (One interesting study in Israel had radiologists attach photos of the patients whose X-rays they were reading to the films. This humanized the experience for them because they could imagine real people with real lives.)
- Try to keep presentations case-based, rather than lecture-style, as this has been shown to motivate physician learning.
- Use the chalkboard or an overhead projector to graph lab results or draw other graphs.

- If a resident is presenting a case or a topic, let her finish with few interruptions, saving questions for the end.
- Summarize key points. Ask Socratic-type questions to stimulate discussion.
- Try to provide handouts, summaries, bibliographies, or review articles at the end of the learning session.

HOW TO GIVE AN EFFECTIVE AUDIOVISUAL PRESENTATION USING POWERPOINT, OVERHEADS, AND SLIDES[5]

- Do not plan to use more than one PowerPoint slide or overhead per minute or you will overwhelm your audience.
- Number and order your slides carefully.
- Use bold print and no more than six lines per slide and six words per line to facilitate reading. Use bullet headings to focus attention.
- Keep graphs and figures simple.
- Consider using dual laptops/projectors to contrast images (e.g., before and after treatment) or text versus an image like a CT scan or X-ray.
- Try not to move backward and forward with slides. If you need to re-reference a slide have another copy of it placed appropriately in your line-up.
- If using a pointer, be incisive to refer to a specific point; don't "wander."

TIP: "I would encourage presenters to remember who their audience is, and what that audience wants to hear vs what the presenter wants to say (with emphasis on the former rather than the latter), and to remember that most people can remember, at best, three key points from a talk. Before I give a talk, I like to ask myself, 'If I could pick one thing for the audience to remember, what would it be?' Then, I try to really hammer that point home and remove unrelated points."

- Bring a back-up memory stick with your presentation material saved to it.
- Arrive in the lecture theater early to set up your laptop and to familiarize yourself with the microphone, audiovisual (AV) equipment, and light dimmer.

- Turn the lights back on during discussion time.
- Pay attention to timing: begin and end your talk promptly in the allotted time, leaving ample time for questions and feedback.
- Remember, you don't always need PowerPoint slides. You can also teach informally ("off the cuff") and encourage dialogue, the sharing of narratives and questions.

Other Tips On Organizing Your Presentation

- State the intent of your talk, outline the learning objectives, and make sure your presentation has a beginning, middle, and end.
- Engage your audience (attention wanes after 15 minutes).
- Keep content relevant, concise, and interesting without too much detail. Use appropriate humor to engage your audience.
- Repeat important take-home messages and summarize.
- Practice speaking clearly in a conversational style with good pacing, volume, and pitch. Don't read a script and, wherever possible, try to interact with your audience.
- Dress professionally for the occasion in comfortable, unrestricting clothing.

BECOMING A LEADER[6]

Being a physician can provide key opportunities to develop your leadership skills.[7] Here are some suggestions from the *CanMEDS Physician Health Guide* for developing your leadership skills:

Much has been written about leadership and how it influences us as individuals and as a society. Many of us need leaders to give us a sense of direction, stability, purpose, and hope. Others do not gravitate toward leaders, maintaining their identity more autonomously. And then there are those who thrive by leading.

In general, leaders are average people who differ from their peers in some ways and mirror them in others. These are people who were born with an innate set of talents and skills (not as common as one might think) and or who grew to develop such a portfolio over time. Regardless of their nature or nurture, leaders have a clear sense of their values and beliefs, have the social skills to attract and maintain relationships with others in a way that motivates action on those values and beliefs, and maintain a transparency, integrity, and genuineness that foster the trust of those who choose to follow.

How do you become a leader? Leadership can be demonstrated in any sphere of action, and on any scale, to bring about positive change and promote improved outcomes. For residents, the acquisition of leadership skills is an important aspect of their development as medical professionals. The following discussion explores a set of catch-phrases that can inspire the cultivation of leadership skills among new physicians.

Get involved. Many organizations could use your energy, ideas, and vision. Your program and its host university will have committees that welcome, and need, resident input; your provincial housestaff organization (PHO) is managed and led by residents and would welcome your input with open and grateful arms; your provincial or state medical association welcomes and needs resident input; and your national organizations (Canadian Association of Internes and Residents, AMA Resident and Fellow Section, the Committee of Interns and Residents [CIR], and your specialty society) have roles and purposes for resident input. You can also partner with international development agencies to offer your skills abroad, or consider working with Médecins Sans Frontières after graduation. All these organizations offer opportunities to put your ideas and personality to the test with lots of support, encouragement, and, in many cases, formal training.

Many organizations outside of medicine would also welcome your input and energy. Habitat for Humanity, Big Brothers/Big Sisters, the United Way, political parties, and non-governmental organizations also present opportunities for leadership development and for personal and professional growth.

Get passionate. Reflect for a while on your core values and beliefs: What is it that most creates energy or tension within you? Perhaps you are a passionate defender of socialized medicine. Perhaps you are a proponent of greater privatization. Perhaps you have a new idea that merits attention. Seek out the people and organizations who would appreciate your contribution and leadership. If a cause puts a fire in your belly, it will sustain your ability to lead. And so, identify your passions and get busy.

Get goal-oriented. Spreading yourself too thin will produce mediocre results. Pick one or two areas of leadership and apply yourself to them as best you can. Not only will this help you maintain balance in your life, it will also help you succeed in those things that you choose to take on. Be a finisher. Leaders didn't get to where they are by stopping halfway down the track.

Get honest and real. Get to know yourself really well. Most leaders can readily identify their critical strengths as perceived by themselves and others. They can also readily identify their vulnerabilities, flaws, and shortcomings – again, as perceived by themselves and others. Be yourself and be genuine: superficiality and phoniness are easy for others to detect. Learn to be comfortable in your own skin, how to use your own strengths and talents, and how to adapt your style of interpersonal engagement to meet the needs of others and the situation at hand.

Get trained. Leadership skills develop over time. Most successful leaders had the benefit of some form of formal leadership training. Typically, leadership courses offer assessment of personality traits and interpersonal styles as part of their curriculum. This process, although sometimes a little painful, is well worth the investment of time and course fees. Ask your provincial or national housestaff and medical associations for their recommendations for leadership training, and also consider opportunities such as the Royal College's *Annual Resident Leadership Program* and the CMA's *Physician-Manager Institute*, which is open to residents from both sides of the border. The AMA offers Executive Leadership programs as well. You can also encourage your program director to develop a local leadership program as part of the core curriculum.

Get ready to learn from mistakes. As you develop leadership skills you will make mistakes. Despite your best intentions, you will bruise feelings, leave people out, subvert processes, create unintentional consequences, and perhaps even do harm. Seek lots of feedback on your leadership efforts, learn the techniques of reflective practice, and develop a process of modifying your own leadership strategies as you move forward.

Get a board of directors. Leaders identify mentorship as one of the most critical elements of a successful career. Everyone benefits from mentorship and by mentoring others. In general, mentors are individuals who negotiate a relationship that focuses primarily on the growth and development of the less experienced of the pair; and some mentors actively seek ways to promote the career development of their mentee. These relationships can be incredibly satisfying and often last for many years.

Indeed, some people have a number of mentors, each of whom helps with a particular area of development (e.g., one for clinical research, one for grant writing, etc.). This collection of experts can be your personal "board of directors" and can enrich your career and life development.

Get the link between leadership and physician health. Leadership development is a tremendous opportunity to focus on your own resiliency. The insights gained in leadership development, particularly with respect to identifying your core values and beliefs, your interpersonal style, and your personality traits, are powerful and practical. When things are stressful and difficult, and your vulnerabilities become apparent, your leadership skills and traits can help you to cope well. In addition, your leadership skills can help promote a system of medicine that enhances the health and well-being of all involved, including all health professionals as well as the patients and families they serve.

(Reprinted, with permission, from Puddester D, *CanMEDS Physician Health Guide*, Ottawa, Royal College of Physicians and Surgeons of Canada, 2009; for more info, check out the RCPSC international resident leadership summit, at http://www.royalcollege.ca/portal/page/portal/rc/events/icre/irls)

What about the Hidden Curriculum?

Few residents and other medical trainees are encouraged to question the wisdom or legitimacy of what they are asked to learn. Curricula are (after all) designed by senior faculty and overseen by licensing bodies, specialty organizations, colleges and institutions, and provide "standards of practice." Most of us refer to "The (official) Curriculum" as the formal, stated, and intended body of knowledge we are all meant to master. This is the actual course of study, and consists of teaching, evaluation of teaching methods, syllabi, and other material used in any educational setting from lecture halls to labs, to seminar rooms, the bedsides, and clinics. The Informal (or delivered) Curriculum is "what actually happens." As Delese Wear of NEOMED reminds us, it consists of "idiosyncratic, popup, and often unplanned instruction that takes place between anyone who is teaching (attendings, residents, or other healthcare professionals) and trainees. It reflects what teachers believe trainees should acquire in terms of knowledge, skills, values, and attitudes."[8]

The Hidden Curriculum, in contrast, involves what is taught inadvertently. This concept originally comes from the educational rather than the medical literature, and it contains messages both ideological and subliminal from the formal and informal curricula. The hidden curriculum is transmitted by individual human behaviors, but also by the structures and practices of institutions, including hospitals and universities. Dr Fred Hafferty, who first applied notions of the hidden curriculum to medicine, described it as "understandings, customs, rituals, and taken-for-granted aspects of what goes on in the life-space we call medical education." It thus consists of unexamined assumptions, values, rules, protocols, privileges, manifestations of power and domination, practices, messages, indifferences to inequity, use of language, and prioritization of what is important and less important in the knowledge to be transmitted.

TIP: *"If possible, it is helpful to continue to read a newspaper, news website, or non-medical magazine to keep up with the world outside of medicine. If nothing else, it helps us relate to our patients. Some suggestions:* Globe and Mail, New York Times, Economist, New Yorker, Harper's, Bloomberg Businessweek, London Telegraph."

Residents often have trouble defining the Hidden Curriculum, but they generally do not have difficulty identifying it when they encounter it. The Hidden Curriculum manifests through negative role modeling, unprofessional behavior, and the message "Do what I say and not what I do" from preceptors and supervisors. In the face of the Hidden Curriculum, learners feel discomfort as their experiences are discounted, and they may feel silenced or powerless in the face of power inequities.

There are some questions to help you discuss how the Hidden Curriculum manifests and plays out in your own learning environment:

1 How do we know what we know? What material is included and what is excluded in what we are taught? (The latter is often referred to as the "Null Curriculum")?
2 How does power play out in any encounter between learner and teacher, doctor and patient? What is the pecking order in this service/ward/clinic?

3   When have I felt discounted, silenced, or ridiculed in my training? How does this represent a microcosm of the overall learning environment?

4   What gets labeled as important in teaching versus "soft," "touchy-feely," or dispensable?

5   How do institutional policies, assessment techniques, and the language we use (including disparaging slang or jargon) illustrate the hidden curriculum?

6   How are my own values challenged by the values of my institution?

7   How has unprofessional behavior been manifested by powerful individuals and then addressed by my institution?

8   What messages about race, class, gender, sexuality, physical ableness, and privilege are given explicitly, implicitly, or in a contradictory manner?

9   How does our current curriculum model societal expectations, rules, inequities, and power structures? Who has a voice and who doesn't?

10   What are examples of hypocrisy and mixed messages in my learning? How are these addressed?

11   What attitudes would I like to see changed in my learning group, class, residency program, profession? How are time and space allocated to particular themes and subject matter, and how does this illustrate the importance or non-importance of these subjects?

12   How is money spent at my institution? How does that suggest what is important?

13   How are dissent, feedback, and helpful criticism handled in my learning environment?

THE REAL WORLD

One of the first clinics I went to in medical school was with an internist locally famous for his diagnostic skills. People said he'd read every issue of *NEJM* cover to cover. And unsurprisingly, he started the observership by pulling a sheaf of photographs from an envelope and asking me to identify the physical findings in each one. Each picture was followed by a question about the physiology of the disease.

But on our way down the hall to see his first patient, the questions changed.

"Who was Madoff?" he asked.

"Sorry, what?" I asked. I couldn't think of a Madoff's sign or any appropriate medical eponym.

"Madoff," he repeated. "The financier who took everyone's money."

And then, later. "Who is Dennis Kucinich?"

This time I was prepared, albeit puzzled.

"You must learn all of Harrison's," he told me afterward, "but it is not enough. Your patients do not read medical textbooks, and if you cannot relate to them, you will never take a good history."

I've noticed this many times since. The best clinicians I've ever met are often the ones with the broadest interests: the old internist who quoted TS Eliot on the wards, or the generalist who stopped me before we went into a patient's room so that we could watch the patient through the window, saying, "Come, Dr Watson. Let us observe."

EXPANDING YOUR WORLDVIEW

No matter what your specialty, increasing your knowledge of cultural and psychosocial issues can only help you become a more consummate healer who provides optimal, person-centered care. Consult an up-to-date psychiatry or behavioral medicine textbook or do a Medline search on the following topics. Incorporate these subjects into rounds, teaching, and case management. Invite guest consultants to discuss them as well. Explore the arts and humanities to broaden your worldview about human experience and suffering. Read broadly as the above resident narrative suggests! They help us challenge assumptions and biases while providing an aesthetic and often provocative experience.

Topics Related to Psychosocial and Cultural Issues

ALL doctors should develop basic, essential skills for treating people living with acute or chronic mental illness and then working with/caring for them over time as part of an engaged, "shared care" team. As you become more experienced, you'll see that arbitrarily or dismissively separating mind from body and mental illnesses from physical illnesses does a huge disservice to our patients and to ourselves as humanistic practitioners.

Aboriginal/Indigenous health
Advocacy
Alcohol and substance abuse
Alternative therapies
Anxiety
Arts for health (i.e., music/art therapies)
Attention deficit, enuresis, and other childhood problems
Body image/"body fascism"
Brief psychotherapy
Child and sexual abuse
Compliance and noncompliance with treatment (now called Adherence)
Corrections facilities and prison healthcare
Cost-benefit decision analysis
Cultural aspects of care
Death and dying
Dementia
Depression and bipolar disorder
"Difficult" patients
Disability studies
The doctor–patient relationship
Drug abuse

Eating disorders
Empathy
End-of-life care and decisions
Epidemiology
Environmental/ecological crises
Ethical issues in care, including euthanasia and physician-assisted suicide
Family violence
Gay and lesbian, bisexual, and transgendered health issues
Gender issues in medical care
Geriatric care
Grief and mourning
HIV-AIDS – medical and psychosocial care
Illness behaviors
Inter-professional studies/ practices
Insomnia
Leadership
Life-cycle issues
Medical and health humanities
Medicare/"Obamacare"/ disability insurance/universal healthcare

Multiculturalism	Professionalism/un-
Narrative in medicine	professional behavior
Obsessive-compulsive	Psychiatric emergencies
disorders	Psychiatry and medicine (models
Occupational health	of collaborative/shared care)
Pain diagnosis and	Psycho-geriatrics
management	Rural /northern medicine
Palliative care	Schizophrenia
Patient safety/clinical error	Sexual assault
Personality disorders	Sexual dysfunction
Pharmaceutical industry	Smoking cessation
practices	Social justice
Phobias	The social sciences and health
Population/minority health	Spousal abuse (male and female)
Power and authority in care	Stigma
and learning	Stress management
Prayer and healing	Suicide
Pregnancy	Women's health and health
Prevention (health)	research

The Medical Humanities

(Source: www.health-humanities.com)

Many of the problems faced by residents and fellows in their education revolve around issues that do not get named or discussed. These include the impact of physician encounters on patients and the important role of non-cognitive attributes in future healers, including exploring feelings as a part of learning and tolerating ambiguity and uncertainty. And what about embodied, working definitions of empathy, reflective capacity, cultural sensitivity and diversity, and the hidden curriculum?

The medical humanities, often called "health humanities" to be more inclusive of other professions, have been defined as "an integrated, interdisciplinary philosophical approach to recording and interpreting human experiences of illness, disability, and medical intervention."[9] In short, the medical humanities are expressly concerned with the human side of medicine. They incorporate several fields, including philosophy, history, the arts, literature, anthropology, sociology, and bioethics.

The health humanities encourage a way of thinking, rather than content-based knowledge, as well as critical thinking (the ability to ask "How do I know what I know"?). They help foster narrative competence – the ability to work with stories, to listen optimally, and to co-construct the meaning of illness and healing with patients over time. They foster visual literacy – the ability to work with non-verbal cues – and reflective capacity – the ability to step back and learn from past experience (reflection on action) so that it can be applied in the here and now (in action).

Humanities scholars themselves also benefit from a critical dialogue with their healthcare counterparts. They can be enriched by an ongoing dialogue with colleagues from clinical disciplines by having direct access to clinical teaching settings, which link to their study of critical theory. They can be invited to help shape the discourse around perceptions of health and illness in our learning community and in the society at large. A more central focus of medical humanities is on increasing the role of the humanities in the provision of good patient care.

The result can be a university-wide community of scholars – what I call "medicine watchers" and clinical practitioners from multiple disciplines – who share (or dispute!) contemporary and historical views on human experience, suffering, and dignity.

The offerings by medical/health humanities divisions in medical schools are rich and diverse. They can include watching films, learning to interpret paintings and perform close reading of literary texts, doing reflective and creative writing, keeping a personal reflective portfolio, organizing seminars about the interface between the arts and medicine, and exploring the arts for health movement. They often invite trainees to develop an artistic practice themselves, which can afford new forms of creative expression and reflection, but also encourage learning with BOTH sides of the brain. They come to honor both thoughts and feelings, the subjective and the objective, in their learning process. These endeavors can help reduce the gap between biomedicine, evidence-based medicine, and the human sciences, such as philosophy, history, sociology, and anthropology. They facilitate interdisciplinary and interprofessional teaching and research, model a patient-centered approach to medical care, challenge biomedical arrogance, and equip doctors to meet the moral challenges of practice not covered expressly (or adeptly) by medical education.

Finally, the humanities also help counteract burnout and cynicism. Reflective, creative practitioners take better care of their patients, but they also take better care of themselves, because they have new tools to challenge their assumptions and to sustain their personal values and sense of purpose while providing optimal care.

TIP: *"I am very fond of the 'On Being a Doctor' section in* Annals of Internal Medicine, *and the 'Best of' collections."*

HUMANITIES AND ARTS-BASED LEARNING – SOME RESOURCES

As well as familiarizing yourself with updated psychosocial articles, consider the use of literary classics for learning, as these can facilitate individual reflection and group discussion on ethics issues of care and on the complexity of human relationships. They can also inoculate you against cynicism about the profession.

Here are some seminal books on what it means to be a doctor and on how history has shaped our profession:

A Short History of Medicine – E. Ackerknecht
*Toward an Aesthetic Medicine: Developing a Core Medical Humanities
    Undergraduate Curriculum* – A. Bleakley, R. Marshall, and
    R. Broemer
The Making of Modern Medicine: Turning Points in the Treatment of Disease
    – M. Bliss
Histoire de médicine et la chirurgie de la grande peste à nos jours –
    P. Boussel
Stories of Sickness – H. Brody
The Healing Art: A Doctor's Black Bag of Poetry – R. Campo
ABC of Learning and Teaching in Medicine – P. Cantillon (ed.)
Doctoring: The Nature of Primary Care Medicine – E.J. Cassell
The Nature of Suffering and the Goals of Medicine – E.J. Cassell
Narrative Medicine: Honoring the Stories of Illness – R. Charon

Stories Matter: The Role of Narrative in Medical Ethics – R. Charon and N. Montello

Final Exam: A Surgeon's Reflections on Mortality – P.W. Chen

This Side of Doctoring: Reflections from Women in Medicine – E.L. Chin

The Call of Stories – R. Coles

The Picture of Health: Medical Ethics and the Movies – H. Colt, S. Quadrelli, and F. Lester

Medicine in the Twentieth Century – R. Cooter and J. Pickstone

Disability Study Reader – L. Davis

History of Medicine – J. Duffin

The Wounded Soldier – A. Frank

Better: A Surgeon's Notes on Performance – A. Gawande

The Checklist Manifesto: How to Get Things Right – A. Gawande

Complications: A Surgeon's Notes on an Imperfect Science – A. Gawande

The Yellow Wallpaper – C.P. Gilman

Narrative Based Medicine: Dialogue and Discourse in Clinical Practice – T. Greenhalgh and B. Hurwitz

The Anatomy of Hope: How People Prevail in the Face of Illness – J. Groopman

How Doctors Think – J. Groopman

Doctors' Stories: The Narrative Structure of Medical Knowledge – K. Montgomery Hunter

A History of Medicine – B. Inglis

Body Language – N. Jain, D. Coppcock, and S.B. Clark

Medical Thinking: A Historical Preface – L.S. King

The Illness Narratives: Suffering, Healing and the Human Condition – A. Kleiman

Medicine: An Illustrated History – A.A. Lyons

Body of Work: Meditations on Mortality from the Human Anatomy Lab – C. Montross

Incidental Findings: Lessons from My Patients in the Art of Medicine – D. Ofri

Singular Intimacies: Becoming a Doctor at Bellevue – D. Ofri

The Courage to Teach – P.J. Palmer

The Greatest Benefit to Mankind – R. Porter

On Doctoring: New, Revised and Expanded Third Edition – R. Reynolds and J. Stone

The Doctor Stories – R. Selzer
Letters to a Young Doctor – R. Selzer
The Development of Modern Medicine: An Interpretation of the Social and Scientific Factors Involved – R. Shryock
Empathy and the Practice of Medicine: Beyond Pills and the Scalpel – H. Spiro, E. Peschel, M.G. Curnen, and D. St James
Literature and Medicine: An Annotated Bibliography – J. Trautman and C. Pollard
Bedside Manners: One Doctor's Reflections on the Oddly Intimate Encounters between Patient and Healer – D. Watts
Teaching during Rounds: A Handbook for Attending Physicians and Residents – D. Weinholts and J. Edwards. The Doctor Stories – W.C. Williams and R. Coles

Journals of the Medical Arts and Humanities

Here are some journals that explore what makes medicine an art.

Ars Medica: A Journal of Medicne, The Arts, and Humanities
　www.ars-medica.ca
Bellevue Literary Review
　www.blreview.org
The Healing Muse
　www.upstate.edu/bioethics/thehealingmuse
Hospital Drive
　http://news.med.virginia.edu/hospitaldrive/
Journal of Medical Humanities
　www.springer.com
Literature and Medicine
　www.muse.jhu.edu/journals/literature_and_medicine/
Medical Education www.mededuc.com
Medical Humanities (BMJ)
　www.mh.bmj.com
Pulse: Voices from the Heart of Medicine
　www.pulsemagazine.org

Films and Videos

Films provide a great medium for sparking discussion and personal reflection about the work we do and how illness and medicine are perceived culturally. Here are some classic films and videos to facilitate group discussion of physician identity and the doctor–patient relationship.

- *And the Band Played On*
- *Article 99*
- *Awakenings*
- *Breaking the Waves*
- *Celebration (Festen)*
- *The Citadel*
- *Cleo from 5:00–7:00*
- *Common Threads: Stories from the AIDS Quilt*
- *Dancer in the Dark*
- *Death of a Salesman*
- *Death Takes a Holiday*
- *The Doctor*
- *The Elephant Man*
- *Frances*
- *Happiness*
- *Hospital*
- *Ikira*
- *I Never Promised You a Rose Garden*
- *Kingdom*
- *The Last Angry Man*
- *Lorenzo's Oil*
- *The Lost Weekend*
- *Magnificent Obsession*
- *Magnolia*
- *Marnie*
- *M*A*S*H*
- *Murmur of the Heart*
- *My Left Foot*
- *One Flew Over the Cuckoo's Nest*
- *Ordinary People*
- *Philadelphia*
- *The Prince of Tides*
- *Resurrection*
- *Scenes from Silver Lake*

- *The Snake Pit*
- *Spellbound*
- *Sunday Bloody Sunday*
- *Sybil*
- *Terms of Endearment*
- *White Corridors*
- *Whose Life Is It Anyway?*
- *Wild Strawberries*
- *Wit*

For a wonderful resource matching films and documentaries to specific clinical topics, go to the NYU Literature, Arts and Medicine Database at http://medhum.med.nyu.edu. Residents and students also enjoy discussing episodes of TV shows. Consider using a favorite (or controversial!) episode from *Grey's Anatomy, House, In Treatment, Nurse Jackie*, or *Scrubs*.

Arts and Health/Humanities Organizations

amh.ac.uk/ (Association for Medical Humanities/UK)
www.asbh.org (Amercian Society of Bioethics and Humanities)
Creating Space – an annual pre-conference for the CCME (Canadian Conference on Medical Education)
  www.mededconference.ca
  www.health-humanities.com

REFERENCES

1 Ellaway R. eMedical Teacher. *Med Teach.* 2011;33(3):258–260. http://dx.doi.org/10.3109/0142159X.2011.561696.
2 Audet N. How to manage CME reading time efficiently. *Can J CME.* 1995(Sept):83–8.
3 Mazmanian PE, Davis DA. Continuing medical education and the physician as learner: Guide to the evidence. *JAMA.* 2002;288(9):1057–60. http://dx.doi.org/10.1001/jama.288.9.1057.
4 Thomson P. Medical education vs. medical educators. *The New Physician,* 2009. http://www.amsa.org/publications/the-new-physician/

5 Snell L. How to give an effective audiovisual presentation. *Can J Contin Med Educ.* 1994(Sept):1–3.

6 Tomlinson C, Labossiere J, Rommens K, et al. The Canadian general surgery resident: Defining current challenges for surgical leadership. *Can J Surg.* 2012;55(4):S184–90.

7 Taylor B. *Effective Medical Leadership.* Toronto: University of Toronto Press; 2010.

8 Wear D, Skillicorn J. Hidden in plain sight: The formal, informal, and hidden curricula of a psychiatry clerkship. *Acad Med.* 2009;84(4):451–8. http://dx.doi.org/10.1097/ACM.0b013e31819a80b7.

9 Evans M. Reflections on the humanities in medical education. *Med Educ.* 2002;36(6):508–13.

CHAPTER NINE

Not Just a Job: Professionalism, Ethics Issues, and Legal Considerations

In 1996 the Royal College of Physicians and Surgeons of Canada introduced an innovative framework called CanMeds for medical education, which established core competencies for all doctors. Seven key roles of the doctor were identified:[1]

- Medical expert
- Communicator
- Collaborator
- Health advocate
- Manager
- Scholar
- Professional

(A new version of CanMeds was released in 2015 and replaced the Manager category with that of Leadership: www.royalcollege.ca/canmeds/canmeds2015)

The Royal College and the College of Family Physicians of Canada defined the "Professional" role as follows:

> Physicians are committed to the health and well-being of individuals and society through ethical practice, profession-led regulation, and high personal standards of behavior. Physicians have a unique societal role as professionals who are dedicated to the health and caring of others. Their work requires the mastery of a complex body of knowledge and skills, as well as the art of medicine. As such, the Professional Role is guided by codes of

ethics and a commitment to clinical competence, the embracing of appropriate attitudes and behaviors, integrity, altruism, personal well-being, and to the promotion of the public good within their domain. These commitments form the basis of a social contract between a physician and society. Society, in return, grants physicians the privilege of profession-led regulation with the understanding that they are accountable to those served.[1]

The Royal College also identified the following key competencies related to professionalism:[1]

- The ability to demonstrate a commitment to patients, the profession, and society through ethical practice
- The ability to demonstrate a commitment to patients, the profession, and society through participation in profession-led regulation
- The ability to demonstrate a commitment to physician health and sustainable practice

The ACGME (Accredited Council for Graduate Medical Education) has also identified core competencies for residents:

- Patient care
- Medical knowledge
- Practice-based learning and improvement
- Interpersonal and communication skills
- Systems-based practice and professionalism

For this last competency, residents must demonstrate a commitment to carrying out professional responsibilities and an adherence to ethical principles. Residents are expected to demonstrate:

- Compassion, integrity, and respect for others;
- Responsiveness to patient needs that supersedes self-interest;
- Respect for patient privacy and autonomy;
- Accountability to patients, society, and the profession; and
- Sensitivity and responsiveness to a diverse patient population, including but not limited to diversity in gender, age, culture, race, religion, disabilities, and sexual orientation.

(Source: https://www.acgme.org/outcome/comp/comphome.asp)

In the 1990s the American Board of Internal Medicine (ABIM) commenced a similar project to advance the evaluation of professionalism as a fundamental component of clinical competence. This subcommittee defined professionalism as "the attitudes and behaviors that serve to maintain patients" interests above physician self-interest.[2] Professionalism aspires to altruism, accountability, excellence, duty, service, honor, integrity and respect for others. The ABIM developed a superb online curriculum including case vignettes, strategies for fostering and evaluating professional attitudes, signs of unprofessionalism, and a comprehensive bibliography (www.abim.org).

Finally, the following statement, published in JAMA, elegantly defines the patient-physician covenant and how it must be guided by both professional and ethical principles:[3]

Medicine is, at its center, a moral enterprise grounded in a covenant of trust. This covenant obliges physicians to be competent and to use their competence in the patient's best interests. Physicians, therefore, are both intellectually and morally obliged to act as advocates for the sick wherever their welfare is threatened and for their health at all times.

Today, this covenant of trust is significantly threatened. From within, there is growing legitimation of the physician's materialistic self-interest; from without, for-profit forces press the physician into the role of commercial agent to enhance the profitability of healthcare organizations. Such distortions of the physician's responsibility degrade the physician–patient relationship that is the central element and structure of clinical care. To capitulate to these alterations of the trust relationship is to significantly alter the physician's role as healer, carer, helper, and advocate for the sick and for the health of all.

By its traditions and very nature, medicine is a special kind of human activity – one that cannot be pursued effectively without the virtues of humility, honesty, intellectual integrity, compassion, and effacement of excessive self-interest. These traits mark physicians as members of a moral community dedicated to something other than its own self-interest.

Our first obligation must be to serve the good of those persons who seek our help and trust us to provide it. Physicians, as physicians, are not, and must never be, commercial entrepreneurs, gate-closers, or agents of fiscal policy that runs counter to our trust. Any defection from primacy of the patient's well-being places the patient at risk by treatment that may compromise quality of or access to medical care.

We believe the medical profession must reaffirm the primacy of its obligation to the patient through national, state, and local professional societies; our academic, research, and hospital organizations; and especially through personal behavior. As advocates for the promotion of health and support of the sick, we are called upon to discuss, defend, and promulgate medical care by every ethical means available. Only by caring and advocating for the patient can the integrity of our profession be affirmed. Thus we honor our covenant of trust with patients.[3]

REFLECTIVE CAPACITY AND PROFESSIONALISM

The fostering of reflective capacity within medical education is recommended to help develop critical thinking skills, inform clinical reasoning, and enhance professionalism. Reflective capacity can be defined as "a critical analysis of knowledge and experience to achieve deeper meaning and understanding." It guides future behavior and is deemed an essential characteristic of professionally competent clinical practice. More recently, reflective capacity has been described as integral to the promotion of professional and ethical core competencies in medical and other clinical practice. Reflection plays an essential role in fostering mindfulness and a sense of integrity and humanism with which to approach clinical reasoning and patient care dilemmas that may arise. There are lots of ways to reflect: mindfulness, meditation, Balint groups, supervision. The usefulness of a reflective writing modality (a subset of narrative-based medicine), in teaching and learning is well documented. (See chapter 13 for recommended readings for this chapter.)

Using Reflective Writing: Ten Tips for Writing and Sharing Personal Narratives

Clinical educators are increasingly asking residents to use writing as a tool for enhancing self-awareness and reflective capacity. Critical incident reports, parallel charts, portfolio entries, and journaling have all been used with success in facilities across North America and are on example of successfully incorporating the humanities into curricula.

Generally, a writing prompt is provided and you'll be asked to either write onsite (for 5 to 20 minutes) or take the prompts home and bring your writings to the next meeting for small-group discussion, formal Portfolio course credit, and feedback. I have been using writing prompts based on CanMEDS professional roles in a new writing elective for clerks at the University of Toronto. The following guidelines derived from that experience may be helpful for residents and educators wishing to use reflective writing in a small-group teaching context.

1 Establish ground rules for the group. Emphasize confidentiality. Some of these stories may be self-revelatory or based on encounters with real patients and colleagues. "What's told in the group stays in the group." Define boundaries. This is a not psychotherapy group. If a resident reads a piece, she/he should be in control of what they wish to reveal at all times. Colleagues may ask questions about the story, but it's always up to the volunteering reader whether they answer or reveal more.

2 Create a safe space for learning and exploration. Tips for giving feedback on writing should be provided. Each reading should be voluntary. The strengths of the piece should always be discussed first – what was moving, powerful, and resonant. Residents may make helpful suggestions on the piece, but the goal is to be constructive and supportive. Even if readers disagree with the sentiment or viewpoint of the piece, their goal is to work with the text itself rather than challenge the author personally.

3 Suggest that residents write about real life, personal incidents – something specific that actually happened. Invite them to write the story as if they were telling a friend and not worry about grammar, spelling, or syntax in the first draft. Encourage them to structure the story with a beginning, middle, and end, and to include how they felt about the incident (not just the facts).

4 Provide short, simple writing prompts that capture the imagination, rather than eliciting intellectualized content or formal essays, such as "Write about a goodbye." Remind residents that prompts are merely a suggested launching pad and that they are free to write about whatever they like.

TIP: *"It's worth reflecting on the true source of stress. People often get upset at patients or other trainees when they are really upset about systems issues (e.g., pressure to admit or discharge, pressure to cover calls)."*

5 When a resident reads a piece to the group, ask them to read the story as written from start to finish (no apologies, explanation, or preamble). Ask them to remain silent during the feedback from the other students so that they can take it all in. Then invite them to rejoin the discussion. They may be surprised by some of the interpretations of their piece, and answering questions or commencing right after reading could hamper that process from unfolding.

6 Ask questions to deepen reflection: "Why did you write this piece and/or choose that incident?" "Did anything surprise you in writing it?" "Would you do anything differently?" "What do you like about your piece?" "What did you struggle with?" "How does it relate to other things you've written?" "Do any learning points emerge for you?"

7 Even though residents may not read to the Reflection/Portfolio group every week, encourage them to write every week even if just for themselves. We suggest taking up to 45 minutes for writing a piece, so that the task doesn't feel onerous or overly time consuming. Learners can take longer if they like.

8 When residents write about patients, remind them that clinical stories are always co-constructed and do not belong to the physician writer alone. They can be shared in a respectful manner for learning and reflection (as in case presentations), but permission should be obtained from the patient if the piece is to be published (including, of course, being posted on a blog).

9 Teachers or senior residents supervising groups should be ready to intervene if a colleague reveals distressing content (i.e., issues related to abuse, self-harm, or professional-boundary violations). A private discussion at the end of the teaching session should be offered and resources for help provided.

10 After the class is finished, encourage your residents to continue writing throughout their career as an ongoing form of personal

reflection. Tell them to keep track of all their "firsts" in medical training – their first delivery, the first death of a patient, their first mistake, their first attempt at a new procedure. Remind them to keep their pieces together so that nothing is lost.

Reflective writing honors both the subjective and objective faces of experience and learning and allows us to document our evolution as human beings and as healers over time.

For more writing prompts and writing tips see:

Allan Peterkin, *Portfolio to Go: 1000 Prompts and Provocations for Clinical Learners* (University of Toronto Press, forthcoming 2016)

ETHICS VS LEGAL CONSIDERATIONS

Medical residents have growing concerns about the risks of litigation during or after their training, and understandably seek ways to protect themselves. Educators in medical ethics and professionalism suggest that this focus is sadly misplaced and that residents should concentrate on learning ethical ways to preserve their relationships with patients and to act in their best interests as professionals. Because ethics and legal principles naturally overlap, it is generally assumed that the ethical physician should rarely be sued, although the application of the law to specific issues and case dilemmas can vary among provinces and states.

Most residents have taken courses and discussed ethics as undergraduates, but formal learning about ethics and professionalism during residency varies considerably from program to program.[4] As well, undergraduate teaching may not prepare them for the "hidden curriculum," where mixed messages about ethical positions, patient care, and collegial relationships conflict with official statements and orthodox messages about professionalism.[5] Because residents make decisions about ethics and physician–patient relationships daily, the lack of formal help or instruction in these areas can add further stress to resident life. Trainees face conflict when they try to respect patients' autonomy if they believe that their own is compromised. (Conversely, they like it when patients readily agree, and this at times may benefit the doctor more than the patient.) Residents whose views differ from those of their patients or who witness malpractice will experience dissonance and confusion. Ethical disagreements with attending physicians, particularly concerning overtreatment, often are not voiced, and this represents a significant stressor.[6] Residents sometimes perform treatment as mandated by superiors, even if they strongly disagree, which causes significant moral distress. Always pay attention to times where you've felt silenced or coerced and reflect on what you did in the acute situation, then identify specific options/solutions for the next time this happens.

This chapter is intended to sensitize you to ethics issues and legal considerations and is designed to allow you to contemplate your role as a medical professional. It is by no means a comprehensive summary of the issues, nor does it offer legal directives. Further resources are provided at the end of this chapter.

ETHICS ISSUES

The DeCamp Foundation recommends that, during postgraduate training, residents should acquire ethics skills related to the following:[7]

- Moral aspects of medical practice
- Informed-consent process
- Patient refusal of treatment
- Management of the incompetent patient (or the patient lacking capacity)
- Withholding of information
- Confidentiality
- Management of the patient with a poor prognosis
- Management of medical resources

You should reflect on the following summary of views on these matters[8–11] during your training in any specialty, seeking supervision when appropriate. Always distinguish what is expedient for the doctor/system from what is good for the patient. Remember that decisions/actions deemed "legal" are not always ethical.

Moral Aspects of Medical Practice

Residents often experience conflict between their wish to heal ("benef-icence") and patients' wish for autonomy and self-determination. In addition, residents' views of illness and of cultural or moral issues may differ dramatically from those of patients. Residents must learn to recognize these inner conflicts and how they relate to the patient, and to ascertain, and then respect, the patient's wishes, rather than adopt an authoritarian, omnipotent stance. If residents cannot appre-ciate a patient's position, either they should say so, explaining what this may mean to their physician–patient contract, or they should help the patient find alternative care. They then remain responsible for their patient's care until another physician is found.

Informed-Consent Process

Informed consent exists to protect the patient, not the hospital or the caregiver. It consists of three key elements:

1 Information must be provided to the patient about the treat-ment or procedure, its purpose, risk–benefit ratio, alternatives, and expected results. Pertinent details must not be withheld because of the physician's wish to obtain consent (often in a hurried state).

2 Comprehension by and capacity of the patient must be assured. Facts must be explained in clear, everyday language with no jargon.

3 Consent must be voluntary – that is, the physician states his or her opinion or position, but does not coerce the patient into making a decision. It is important to keep in mind that "blanket consent" given by the patient on entering hospital is not sufficient. Consent must be sought and obtained for each new procedure or change in treatment.

Patient Refusal of Treatment

A patient has the right to refuse treatment if his reason is adequately explored and is not based solely on misunderstanding, misinforma-tion (e.g., from physician-patient conflict), or coercion from external sources. The likely consequences of failure to give treatment should be presented to the patient. In most hospitals a patient is then asked to sign a statement affirming that treatment has been refused in full knowledge of these consequences. It is important to remember that this choice should not automatically be equated with incapacity/incompetence or a suicidal tendency in the patient, although these possibilities must be explored. Take the time to find out what the patient's beliefs, fears, concerns, and misperceptions are.

Management of the Patient Who Is Incapable

Incapable/"Incompetent" patients lack the capacity to make decisions about their own care and well-being. They cannot understand information relevant to a decision, consider choices logically, make a choice consistent with their own values, or communicate that choice.[7] Most incapable patients have chronic neurological conditions that affect cognition, insight, and memory, such as dementia or post-stroke or post-traumatic syndromes. Some psychiatric illnesses (like acute psychosis) also affect insight/judgment. Legislation defining who can declare a patient incapable/incompetent varies; in some areas it is any physician, whereas in others it must be a psychiatrist. Chart documentation always includes a mental status exam and a commentary on the three criteria for informed consent (information, comprehension, and voluntariness). Verify the appropriate procedure with the hospital's social services department. Also check to see if the patient had previously completed a living will or advance directive.

If informed consent cannot be given because of a lack of capacity (formerly called "incompetence," a loaded term for many), the resident, with the help of a social worker, will want to initiate the proceedings for naming a substitute decision-maker or healthcare proxy, the details and designations of which vary from province to province and from state to state. The substitute decision-maker or healthcare proxy is an appointed person who must be able to determine what the patient would have wished if able to choose, not what is best for the estate, the family, or the proxy. Ideally, this person is someone who loves and respects the patient and may be a family member, but it cannot be assumed that the spouse or a sibling will best serve the patient's interests.

Withholding of Information

Physicians have traditionally used "therapeutic privilege" to withhold potentially "harmful" or "devastating" information from a patient, often at the request of the family. Today this is seldom deemed appropriate by lawyers and ethics consultants because the competent patient has the right to know about diagnosis, treatment, prognosis, alternatives, and risks. As Perkins[7] has pointed out, the question is not *whether* to tell, but *how* to tell. The physician is ethically bound to convey difficult news compassionately and to deal with the results, while continually offering information and support to the patient.

Confidentiality

The resident should not release information about a patient to anyone without clear authorization or express approval, which should be documented in the chart. This also means not chatting about patients where you might be overheard – in the elevator, hallway, or cafeteria. Caution with respect to protection of and access to medical records must be emphasized to all staff, especially with respect to new technologies, such as computerized records, email, fax machines, and cellular telephones, that may be accessed by unauthorized individuals. "Implied consent" traditionally referred to a physician divulging details about a patient to family members or other members of the treatment team, but even this practice should be explored with the patient and recorded. Residents are often casual in the way they discuss some patients with each other (i.e., in an elevator or in the cafeteria), because of the potential for learning involved or an unconscious need to vent their feelings. This practice is increasingly being viewed as unethical because it may violate a patient's consent about what is said about him or her, and to whom. In the United States, up-to-date information on the Health Insurance Portability and Accountability Act (HIPAA) can be found at www.hhs.gov and www.ama-assn.org. In Canada, information on the Personal Information Protection and Electronic Documents Act (PIPEDA) and other documents related to patient privacy can be found at the office of the Privacy Commissioner of Canada, at www.privcom. gc.ca. New challenges to confidentiality include emails, blogging, and the use of electronic devices. Please see "Digital Professionalism Framework," in chapter 12.

Exceptions to absolute protection of a patient's medical privacy vary locally, but include the following situations:

- A subpoena to give evidence in court (where files and documents can be held as evidence)
- A court order or search permit to produce a patient's chart (not simply a visit from a police officer or sheriff)
- Reporting to appropriate authorities child or elder abuse, gunshot wounds, unsafe drivers and pilots, certain venereal diseases, and workplace accidents
- Reporting to appropriate authorities a patient's imminent danger to self or others (suicide, homicide, rape, kidnapping, violent behavior, etc.)

Management of the Patient with a Poor Prognosis[9]

Every resident during training is faced with decisions about continuing treatment as opposed to palliation and non-resuscitation of terminally ill patients, and must become familiar with making such distinctions. These decisions are often heart-wrenching and difficult. Each institution you work in will have a policy on resuscitation and how to document decision making, so become familiar with it. In Canada and elsewhere, new legislation on the legality of "assisted suicide" in specific situations has become a source of debate and ethical concern for many doctors. General guidelines from various medical, nursing, and hospital associations for non-resuscitation include the following:

- An assessment that the condition is irreversible and estimates of how long the patient might live without intervention, as well as of the consequence of no-code status (i.e., a "do not resuscitate" order)
- An assessment of the patient's competence and ability to understand risks, benefits, consequences, and options with respect to a no-code status
- Consultation with an appropriate family member if the patient is incompetent
- Documentation of the attending physician's approval and a second opinion from another physician or clinical ethics consultant if there is doubt about the suitability of a no-code status
- A clear order written in the chart to clarify the no-code status

Management of Medical Resources

The management of medical resources is a controversial issue beyond the scope of this discussion, and its ramifications differ considerably between socialized medical systems (as in Canada) and private ones (as in the United States, where the American Medical Association has prepared a document called the "AMA Ethical and Judicial Affairs Ethics Guidelines for Managed Care": www.ama-assn.org). The resident should, however, remember the fundamental principle that every human being is entitled to appropriate care, regardless of diagnosis, race, creed, or ability to pay. Residents must be prepared to advocate for patients, which may at times lead to disagreement with supervisors and their hospital hierarchy. Your focus should be on individual patients and bedside decisions rather than macro-level policy making.

Patient Safety – a Top Priority

An increasing and well-placed focus on the comprehensive care of patients looks at errors, safety risks, and best protocols for patient safety.

Researchers from the Rand Corporation, Stanford, UCSF, John Hopkins, the ECRI Institute, and 21 interested stakeholders examined the existing discourse on patient safety and published their finding in 2013. They were able to identify methods of evaluating the effectiveness of patient safety strategies as well as contexts and elements that improve patient safety. Many of these will make perfect sense to you as you learn/order new procedures and complete hospital rotations.

Patient Safety Strategies Ready for Adoption Now

Strongly encouraged

- Preoperative checklists and anesthesia checklists to prevent operative and postoperative events
- Bundles that include checklists to prevent central-line-associated bloodstream infections
- Intervention to reduce urinary catheter use, including catheter reminders, stop orders, or nurse-initiated removal protocols
- Bundles that include head-of-bed elevation, sedation, vacation, oral care with chlorhexidine, and subglotic suctioning endotracheal tubes to prevent ventilator-associated pneumonia
- Hand hygiene

- The do-not-use list for hazardous abbreviations
- Multi-component interventions to reduce pressure ulcers
- Barrier precautions to prevent care-associated infections
- Use of real-time ultrasonography for central line placement
- Interventions to improve prophylaxis for venous thromboembolisms

Encouraged

- Multicomponent interventions to reduce falls
- Use of clinical pharmacists to reduce adverse drug events
- Documentation of patient preferences for life-sustaining treatment
- Obtaining informed consent to improve patients' understanding of the potential risks of procedures
- Team training
- Medication reconciliation
- Practices to reduce radiation exposure from fluoroscopy and CT
- The use of surgical outcome measurements and reports cards, such as those from the American College of Surgeons' National Surgical Quality Improvement Program
- Rapid-response systems
- Use of complementary methods for detecting adverse events or medical errors to monitor for patient safety problems
- Computerized provider order entry
- Use of simulation exercises in patient safety efforts

Source: Shekelle PG, Wachter RM, Pronovost P, Making health care safer II: An updated critical analysis of the evidence for patient safety practices, *Comparative Effectiveness Review*. 2013 Mar; 2.

Learning More about Professionalism and Ethics Issues

The following suggestions are offered for learning more about medical ethics:

- Consult the CanMeds and ABIM websites listed above.
- Request and attend ethics case conferences, grand rounds, lectures, and retreats.

- Arrange debates or seminars around emerging trends/controversies. For example, how will recent Canadian court decisions about the legality of assisted suicide affect your patients, your practice, and your sense of being a doctor?
- Try to incorporate ethics issues into your regular case presentations, or into other residents' discussion groups to stimulate discussion.
- Introduce ethics concerns into daily work. For example, "Should we be having free lunches on behalf of pharmaceutical companies, or is this a conflict of interest?"
- Seek guidance and examples from more senior residents and attending physicians.
- For tips on ethics integration in teaching see Howard F, Integrating bioethics into postgraduate medical education: The University of Toronto model, *Acad Med* 2010; 85(6).
- Consider pursuing a Master's degree or PhD in bioethics during your residency.
- Contact the hospital's ethics consultant about the particular difficulties of a case.
- Pay attention to your own levels of discomfort when you sense something is unethical, and try to discuss these feelings with a colleague. Do not dismiss such feelings or let them add to your anxiety.
- Consult the books by Jonsen[11] and Beauchamp[12] in the References; they are practical, case-oriented pocket guides to medical ethics and legal matters.
- Refer to the CMA's or AMA's Code of Ethics (available online at www.cma.ca, https://www.cma.ca/En/Pages/code-of-ethics.aspx and http://www.ama-assn.org/ama/pub/physician-resources/medical-ethics/code-medical-ethics.page.
- Consider finding and attending an ethics seminar, workshop, or refresher course offered by a university continuing medical education program.
- Prepare a grand rounds on an ethics topic.
- Call the National Reference Center for Bioethics Literature at Georgetown University (1-800-MED ETHX or visit https://www.bioethics.georgetown.edu) for reference help.
- Read broadly to stretch your thinking.

Readings in Medical Ethics

Here is a list from the "Great Books in Medical Ethics" course offered by the Evanston, Illinois, Hospital Department of Medicine. Consider forming a journal club to explore ethical issues raised by these classic literary works (see the last chapter for additional titles):

The Doctor's Dilemma – George Bernard Shaw
The Hippocratic Oath
Cancer Ward – Alexander Solzhenitsyn
The Death of Ivan Illych – Leo Tolstoy
An Enemy of the People – Henrik Ibsen
A Very Easy Death – Simone De Beauvoir
The Plague – Albert Camus
"A Country Doctor " (story) – Franz Kafka
"Ward Six" (story) – Anton Chekhov
Tender Is the Night – F. Scott Fitzgerald
Frankenstein – Mary Shelley
Erewhon – Samuel Butler
The Power and the Glory – Graham Greene
The Imaginary Invalid and The Doctor in Spite of Himself – Molière
Man's Search for Meaning – Victor Frankl
The Elephant Man – Bernard Pomeranz
The Physician in Literature (excerpts) – Norman Cousins
Equus – Peter Shaffer

Hippocratic Oath[13]

[It's interesting to consider this historical document and to compare it with subsequent physician oaths.]

I swear by Apollo, the physician ... that according to my ability and judgment, I will keep this oath and stipulation: to reckon him who taught me this art equally dear to me as my parents, to share my substance with him and relieve his necessities if required; to regard his offspring as on the same footing with my own brothers, and to teach them this art if they should wish to learn it, without fee or stipulation, and that by precept, lecture and every other mode of instruction ...

I will follow that method of treatment which, according to my ability and judgment, I consider for the benefit of my patients, and abstain from whatever is deleterious and mischievous. I will give no deadly medicine to anyone if asked, nor suggest any such counsel; furthermore, I will not give to a woman an instrument to produce an abortion.

With purity and holiness I will pass my life and practice my art. I will not cut a person who is suffering with a stone, but will leave this to be done by practitioners of this work. Into whatever houses I enter I will go unto them for the benefit of the sick and will abstain from every voluntary act of mischief and corruption; and further from the seduction of females or males, bond or free.

Whatever, in connection with my professional practice or not in connection with it, I may see or hear in the lives of men, which ought not be spoken abroad, I will not divulge ...

Hippocrates, 5th century BC

LEGAL CONSIDERATIONS

Although ethically sensitive residents and effective communicators are less likely to be sued successfully, there are, nonetheless, several measures they can take to protect themselves from legal action. Here are a list of the most common allegations leading to medical malpractice suits and strategies for avoiding them:

1 Failure to diagnose or treat
2 Failure to obtain appropriate consultation
3 Improper or inaccurate communication among healthcare workers
4 Unnecessary, improper, or negligent intervention or treatment
5 Failure to respond to patient inquiry or emergent request
6 Untimely or premature discharge from hospital
7 Failure to obtain legal consent (i.e., prior to anesthesia)
8 Equipment malfunction
9 Abandonment or discharge from care without arranging appropriate follow-up or referral

TIP: "I always schedule at least one day off the week after an ICU/CTU rotation to give myself a long weekend if possible."

Table 9.1   Recommendations for Transferring Care

CAIR believes that patient safety can be enhanced by improved handover education. We recommend that:

1 Each patient handover should incorporate direct verbal interaction between care providers. Given the complexity of the handover process, using both verbal and written communication will ensure safe and accurate transfer of patient care.

2 Handover should take place in a quiet area where distractions are minimal. Sufficient time must be allotted for the handover.

3 The handover process should employ evidence-based tools and be standardized for each clinical setting. There are a variety of mnemonics and aids that may be adapted to the particular needs of a clinical setting.

4 A formal handover curriculum should be an accreditation standard for medical education, reflecting the core competencies of the CanMEDS framework.

5 Physicians require both didactic and interactive training in handover. The interactive component is especially important, and supervised evaluation of handover should be part of the training curriculum. A senior or chief resident, faculty member, or program director should regularly observe each resident's handover performance and provide formal feedback.

Avoiding Litigation

There are things you can do to avoid complaints of malpractice. Here are some tips.

- Keep your focus patient-centered and communicate effectively!
- Avoid coercion, misrepresentation of facts, or leaving conflicts unresolved with patients. Address a patient's dissatisfaction openly and calmly (see chapter 6). Physicians with good communication skills and good relationships with their patients are rarely sued, even if they have made an error in judgment.
- If in doubt about a diagnosis, treatment, or procedure in a particular patient's care, always obtain support for your decision from the senior resident, the attending physician, or a consultant. Document this information in the chart. Your residency malpractice insurance or union (housestaff association) guidelines may require you to discuss all aspects of care with your attending physician, but it is particularly important to record this information when discharging patients. Such guidelines may also come from your program and local licensing authority.
- Document all "transfers of care," that is, when signing over post-call, post-shift, or on leaving rotations. Residents worldwide have perfected safety-maximizing protocols for reliable, systematic

transfers of care. See CAIR's Recommendations for Transferring Care (table 9.1; www.residentdoctors.ca). Call your hospital's director of professional services, residency director, union representative, or union lawyer if inadequate supervision or co-coverage is available to you during call or emergency-department duty, and document this exchange.

- If you make an error in an order, treatment, or procedure, do not attempt to hide it. Discuss it directly with the senior resident or attending physician or hospital manager to learn how and when the information should be divulged to the patient and family. Be sincere in your apologies. Do not alter medical records. (The Electronic Medical Record [EMR] will demonstrate/date and time-stamp these attempts in any case.) For useful sample guidelines on disclosing adverse events, go to www.cmpa-acpm.ca and access a checklist on "communicating with your patient about harm."
- Be sure to obtain proper consent from a patient before a procedure or treatment is started. If you do not, you could be charged with assault and battery. Because the attending physician ultimately is responsible for consent if he or she performs the surgery, determine what information he or she wants given and how it should be given.
- Do not release any information to a third party without written, documented consent. Ask the hospital's legal department under what circumstances patients have the right to see their own charts. (Patients should have the right to do so. Usually a physician must be present to explain the aspects of care detailed in the chart so there are no misunderstandings.)
- Always double-check the orders of juniors and medical students before signing them, because you are responsible for the consequences.
- Verify how much your attending physician expects to be involved in patient care and decision making and the kind and frequency of documentation expected from you (e.g., once a week in a rehabilitation setting vs several times a day in an intensive care unit).
- Make sure you have adequate malpractice protection that covers you for the full period of the statute of limitations (the designated number of years a patient can sue a physician after the particular intervention) in your province or state. Investigate whether you are

covered for moonlighting rather than assuming you are insured outside the hospital.

- When preparing written prescriptions, *print* drug names, indications, dosing, and timing instructions. Avoid abbreviations, sloppy handwriting, and vague directions like "prn." When handing a prescription in, spell the patient's name and the drug name carefully.[14] Avoid oral ("verbal") orders, as they put you, patients, and nursing staff at risk. The AMA House of Delegates, in one of its annual meetings, stressed that "medication errors expose patients to additional but preventable risks leading frequently to prolongation of hospital stay and in some cases contributing to morbidity and mortality, medication errors being the most common case of non-op adverse events (19.4%) and the second most prevalent and second most costly reason for medical malpractice litigation" (www.ama-assn.org). Most of us use EMRs and print prescriptions from their database using our office computers. It's still important to double-check the name of the patient with date of birth and the name/dosing of medications on all printed or handwritten prescriptions.
- Maintain good rapport with patients. Avoid making inappropriate or angry comments. Improve cultural sensitivity around ethnic groups.
- Obtain a patient's permission before discussing her care with family members.
- Discuss the benefits, risks, and statistical results of a particular procedure or treatment with your patient, and document the discussion in the chart.
- Date and time all patient visits, orders, and interventions. Document if you were instructed by your senior resident or attending physician.
- Always search and record potential drug contraindications or allergies, or previous drug interactions. Hospital pharmacists can help you with this.
- Keep your charting and dictations up to date.
- Do not agree to partake in research protocols unless they have been cleared by the university and/or hospital ethics committees.
- Verify hospital and local guidelines on curatorship, commitment, use of restraints, and consent issues. Learn whether the age of majority differs from the age of consent to treatment. When a

patient is a legal minor, try to have the patient's consent to notify his or her parents. If the treatment is potentially controversial, you may have to obtain parental or guardian consent yourself. Consider obtaining an external consultation.

- Have controversial and sensitive procedures witnessed (e.g., pelvic exams and procedures such as lumbar puncture post-trauma that may result in complications). Document the name of the attendant.
- Be aware of legally sensitive areas such as rape, child abuse, custody, and potentially violent behavior when interviewing patients.

Review reporting protocols and make sure you prepare very precise documentation because you may have to give evidence in court.

- Request periodic lectures from your hospital's legal department on specific topics that apply not only to residency, but also to eventual hospital or community-based practice.
- Use caution in emailing patients, as confidentiality may be at risk.

Residents may sometimes be asked to testify about patients they have seen, treated, or assessed. Here are several tips for testifying.[15]

- In Canada, call the Canadian Medical Protective Association for guidelines if you are a member. In the United States, speak to your housestaff representative, hospital risk manager, or malpractice insurer.
- Determine whether it would be more appropriate for your attending physician to appear as the person finally responsible for the patient's care.
- Clarify details of your expected appearance (fees, date, time, and location) with the lawyer who has consulted you.
- To avoid wasted time, request that you be called just before your appearance in court and ask whether a detailed written report would be adequate instead of an appearance.
- Discuss with the lawyer who requests your testimony what evidence is expected from you and how to address the judge. Let her know if you have objections to the usual procedure of swearing in witnesses with the Christian Bible.

- Bring copies of reports, X-rays, and other documents, because the originals may be kept as evidence. Be prepared with a brief summary or notes.
- Be prepared to state your credentials; you must establish your credibility and expect to be challenged.
- Stay calm and present a serious demeanor. Do not become angry, irreverent, or comical. Use simple terms and do not bluff if you do not know the answer to a question.
- See the additional resources in chapter 13 for useful references on coping with the severe stresses of litigation.

OATH FOR NEW DOCTORS[16]

I swear to fulfill, to the best of my ability and judgment, this covenant:

I will respect the hard-won scientific gains of those physicians in whose steps I walk, and gladly share such knowledge as is mine with those who are to follow.

I will apply, for the benefit of the sick, all measures which are required, avoiding those twin traps of overtreatment and therapeutic nihilism.

I will remember that there is art to medicine as well as science, and that warmth, sympathy and understanding may outweigh the surgeon's knife or the chemist's drug.

I will not be ashamed to say "I know not," nor will I fail to call in my colleagues when the skills of another are needed for a patient's recovery.

I will respect the privacy of my patients, for their problems are not disclosed to me that the world may know. Most especially must I tread with care in matters of life and death. If it is given me to save a life, all thanks. But it may also be within my power to take a life; this awesome responsibility must be faced with great humbleness and awareness of my own frailty. Above all, I must not play at God. I will remember that I do not treat a fever chart, or a cancerous growth, but a sick human being, whose illness may affect his family and his economic stability. My responsibility includes these related problems, if I am to care adequately for the sick.

I will prevent disease whenever I can, for prevention is preferable to cure. I will remember that I remain a member of society, with social obligations to all my fellow men, those sound of mind and body, as well as the infirm ...

Louis Lasagna, 1964 (see www.aapsonline.org/ethics/oaths.htm)

REFERENCES

1 Royal College of Physicians and Surgeons of Canada. www.royalcollege.ca/portal/page/portal/rc/public.

2 American Board of Internal Medicine. www.abim.org

3 Crawshaw R, Rogers DE, Pellegrino ED, et al. Patient-physician covenant. [Reprinted with permission.] *JAMA*. 1995;273(19):1553. http://dx.doi.org/10.1001/jama.1995.03520430089054.

4 Jacobson JA, Tolle SW, Stocking C, et al. Internal medicine residents' preferences regarding medical ethics education. *Acad Med*. 1989;64(12):760–4. http://dx.doi.org/10.1097/00001888-198912000-00015.

5 Hundert EM, Hafferty F, Christakis D. Characteristics of the informal curriculum and trainees' ethical choices. *Acad Med*. 1996;71(6):624–42. http://dx.doi.org/10.1097/00001888-199606000-00014.

6 Shreves JG, Moss AH. Residents' ethical disagreements with attending physicians. *Acad Med*. 1996;71(10):1103–5. http://dx.doi.org/10.1097/00001888-199610000-00020.

7 Perkins HS. Teaching medical ethics during residency. *Acad Med*. 1989;64(5):262–6. http://dx.doi.org/10.1097/00001888-198905000-00013.

8 Jonsen AR, Siegler M, Winslade WJ. *Clinical Ethics: A Practical Approach to Decisions in Clinical Medicine*. 7th ed. New York: McGraw-Hill; 2010.

9 Beauchamp TL, McCullough LB. *Medical Ethics: The Moral Responsibilities of Physicians*. Englewood Cliffs, NJ: Prentice-Hall; 1984.

10 Evans KG, Brown NF. *Consent: A Guide for Canadian Physicians*, 4th ed.

11 Evans KG. *Summary of Federal Legislation and Laws Enacted in the Province of Quebec*. Ottawa: CMPA; 1990.

12 Ellaway R. eMedical teacher. *Med Teach*. 2010;32(8):705–7. http://dx.doi.org/10.3109/0142159X.2010.505849.

13 Hutchison R. Do not resuscitate – the writing of no-code orders. *Humane Med*. 1990;6:135–7.

14 *Code of Ethics*. Ottawa: Canadian Medical Association; 2004.

15 Emson H. Testifying. Courtroom etiquette. Here come the judge – are you ready? [*Med Post suppl*] *Curr Ther*. (Seaforth). 1989;(Sept):25–7.

16 Oath for new doctors. *New York Times*, 15 May 1990.

CHAPTER TEN

Taking Care of Business: Managing Your Finances

The complete details of budgeting and investing and of planning and setting up a practice are beyond the scope of this chapter. In Canada, more information can be obtained from the Canadian Medical Association, provincial residency associations, and the MD Management Limited network.[1,2] This network also offers superb tax, financial set-up, and financial counseling seminars, preferred loans, and other services to Canadian medical residents in training. In the United States, the American Medical Association offers some practice-related workshops.[1] Student loan repayment protocols, for example, change over time; they are published in *The Physician's Guide to Financial Planning*. Further financial information can be obtained from unions, the Committee of Interns and Residents (CIR), the American College of Physicians (ACP), the American Association of Medical Colleges (AAMC), the American Medical Students' Association (AMSA), and occasionally at the hospital or state-association program level.

This chapter touches briefly on the following areas: budgeting, education debts, moonlighting and its tax implications, insurance, obtaining loans, and getting help from other professionals. Try to set yourself defined, time-specific goals and then track them over time. Keep all of your documentation organized, up to date, and let your spouse/executor know where your loan, banking, credit card, investment, insurance, and tax information is stored. Check your credit rating at least once a year.

BUDGETING

A budget consists of income and expenses (both fixed and variable). A monthly budget should be updated regularly with your partner and include the following items:

Income Sources

- Salary: own and spouse's
- Pensions
- Bonuses
- Investments: dividends, interest, rent
- Research or other grants
- Alimony
- Child support
- Moonlighting
- Other income

Fixed Expenses

- Housing: mortgage, rent
- Utilities: phone, heat, water, electricity
- Property: taxes, maintenance costs, and insurance
- Healthcare: medical insurance and deductions, medications, dental care, family health coverage
- Loan payback (e.g., on student loans)
- Insurance: life, disability, catastrophic health event policies, malpractice
- Income taxes
- Transportation: public versus own vehicle (insurance, maintenance, licensing, parking)
- Child care
- Board examinations, licensing, professional, and medical society fees
- Other expenses
- You may wish to establish an emergency fund for unforeseen expenses.

Variable Expenses (Areas to Control)

- Conferences/CME/books
- Retirement investment
- Other loans (car, personal, credit cards, line of credit)
- Food
- Household expenses
- Clothing, laundry, cleaning
- Pocket money
- Transportation
- Vacations
- Gifts
- Charities
- Repairs (household)
- Entertainment (concerts, films, clubs, television, publications)
- Emergency funds
- Retirement contributions (start early!)

Table 10.1 Your Net Worth

Assets		
Cash or equivalent		
	Bank accounts, savings	$_____
	Bank accounts, checking	$_____
	Life insurance cash value	$_____
	Other	$_____
Securities		
	Stocks, common and preferred	$_____
	Mutual funds	$_____
	Bonds	$_____
	Other	$_____
Real estate		
	Home	$_____
	Cottage	$_____
	Other buildings	$_____
	Land	$_____
	Other	$_____
Other investments		
	Medical practice	$_____
	Retirement savings plan	$_____
	Home ownership savings plan	$_____
	Other business ventures	$_____

Assets		
Other property		
	Home furnishings (appliances, furniture)	$_____
	Cars	$_____
	Boats, planes, recreational equipment	$_____
	Jewelry, furs	$_____
	Collections (art, stamps, etc.)	$_____
	Other	$_____
Debts owed to you		$_____
Miscellaneous		$_____
Total assets		$_____

Liabilities		
Mortgages outstanding		
	Home	$_____
	Other buildings	$_____
	Land	$_____
	Other	$_____
Loans outstanding		
	Banks, savings and loan	$_____
	Broker	$_____
	Insurance policy loan	$_____
	Other (student)	$_____
	Other	$_____
Taxes		
	Income tax (federal and provincial or state)	$_____
	Property	$_____
	Other	$_____
Bills outstanding		$_____
Miscellaneous		$_____
Total liabilities		$_____
Net worth (assets minus liabilities)		$_____

EDUCATION DEBTS

Some provinces in Canada allow a 6-month grace period after completion of medical school before repayment on government loans is due, but there is some variation. In Quebec, for instance, the grace period is often allowed to continue through residency, which is classified as postgraduate education. The Ontario Medical Students' Association is lobbying for interest-free loan status until the completion of residency training. Check these regulations with your university's registrar, postgraduate medical office, the Canadian Medical Association (www.cma.ca), or an accountant familiar with medical residents' issues.

Education debts can be a source of extreme stress for medical residents in the United States, where traditionally loans had a 2-year interest-deferment period during internship and a 10-year payback limit after completion of medical school. Since residency lasts from 4 to 6 years, these conditions can be a source of considerable stress. (Strikingly, primary care physicians in the first 3–5 years following residency often have expenses that exceed earnings.) Residents can request a forbearance to not make payments during residency, but interest charges will generally start after the 2-year period. AMSA, the CIR, and the American Medical Association have been lobbying effectively to change the legislation governing these conditions including the length of the payback period. (For updates, see the Resident Resource section of the AMA website, www.ama-assn.org, and visit the AAMC loan repayment/foreigners and scholarship website database at www.aamc.org.) In Canada, you may be able to extend your repayment period to a maximum of 19.5 years. It's also essential to investigate debt-repayment incentives offered in underserviced/northern/rural areas in both Canada and the United States.

MEDICAL MOONLIGHTING AND ITS TAX IMPLICATIONS

Moonlighting can provide a lucrative source of added income, but the following factors should be weighed:

- Whether the residency program policies approve of moonlighting; be aware that some programs will undermine your attempts at lobbying to limit residency hours by pointing out that residents voluntarily seek out extra (moonlighting) hours.
- Provincial or state restrictions on moonlighting (e.g., hospital vs outpatient settings, applicable hours); the Accreditation Council for Graduate Medical Education (ACGME), for instance, prohibits work within one period of a regular residency-scheduled shift.

- Whether your malpractice insurance provides coverage outside the hospital and whether the moonlighting establishment will offer such coverage
- The need for and availability of supervision
- Potential scheduling conflicts with residency and home life
- Licensing regulations (i.e., your eligibility to prescribe drugs outside of a training milieu)
- Earnings from fees (your employer will deduct a percentage for overhead from your billing, the rates usually ranging from 25 to 40%)
- Get the overhead rate stated in writing and signed by an authorized official.
- Keep a record of your billings and ask your employer for official receipts.
- Availability of support, secretarial services, and referral sources
- You should not be coerced to do moonlighting; work in the setting where you are actually training.
- Pay attention to your energy levels – do not moonlight if it exhausts you or interferes with study time.

Self-Employed Physicians

Moonlighting will allow you to increase tax deductions and credits because you are a self-employed physician. These deductions and credits can include the following:

- Rent and administration charges
- Salaries and employee benefits
- Medical supplies
- Office taxes and insurance
- Office supplies and expenses
- Office telephones and other equipment
- Medical journals, textbooks
- Office repairs and maintenance
- All other expenses that help you earn income (e.g., cleaning bills)
- Convention expenses
- Continuing medical education expenses
- Entertainment expenses
- Malpractice insurance/CMPA coverage in Canada
- Professional services

- Travel expenses (a percentage of your car expenses related to your practice)
- Office at home
- Interest and bank charges; any interest that you must pay on loans used for business purposes or for earning income and any bank charges related to these loans
- Leasing fees (automobile and equipment)
- Depreciation of furniture and textbooks
- Moving expenses to relocate after residency

OTHER TAX DEDUCTIONS

Your accountant will advise you as to how purchasing government bonds and pension and retirement investment plans (i.e., Registered Retirement Savings Plans in Canada, and Individual Retirement Accounts in the United States) can reduce your tax load.

If you are not moonlighting (i.e., not self-employed), your tax deductions and credits may be limited to the following: tuition, monthly student deduction, equipment and textbooks, exam and insurance fees, and moving expenses (in the first year of residency), besides the standard deductions and credits detailed on tax forms.

Other tax areas to explore with your accountant depend on your particular circumstances and include child care, interest on mortgages (in the United States), investment losses, medical expenses (in excess of a certain percentage of your income), charitable or political donations, sales tax credits, child education plans, and spousal income sharing.

INSURANCE

Make sure you explore and fully consider all insurance options. Check your housestaff agreement for details. Purchase coverage while you're healthy!

Life Insurance Terms and Definitions

- *Whole life*: provides a fixed amount of insurance protection and an accumulation of savings in exchange for a regular premium until the insured's death.

- *Limited payment life*: whole life insurance for which the premiums are level but paid over a specified period (e.g., 20-pay life, single-premium life).
- *Endowment policy*: combines life insurance and savings as in whole life; however, the policy has a specified maturity date – if the policy holder lives to this maturity date, he or she can opt to receive the face value as a lump sum or to receive payments for life or over a specified number of years.
- *Critical life*: covers you for acute/new onset life-threatening illnesses (as delineated in the contract) and offers a lump-sum for those conditions.
- *Participating*: policy holders are given a share in the total profitability of the insuring company; this is commonly called a dividend, but is in reality a refund on premium overpayments.
- *Non-participating*: policy holders have no rights to share in the profits of the company; the premium is fixed and is calculated on the basis of an estimate of interest rates, administration costs, and future mortality.
- *Double indemnity*: the beneficiary receives twice the face value of the policy if the insured's death is the result of an accident.
- *Term (or temporary) insurance*: called "pure protection" because it has no cash-surrender or loan value; policies are insured for specified periods, and benefits are paid only if death occurs within the term of the policy.
- *Level term*: the face value remains constant over the life of the policy.
- *Decreasing term*: the face value of the policy decreases each year, but the premium remains the same.
- *Renewable term*: can be renewed after a prescribed period of time.
- *Convertible term*: may be converted to permanent coverage within a prescribed period without evidence of insurability.

Most residents in Canada and the United States are provided a combination of life, health, and disability insurance through their hospitals, housestaff unions, or university. Ask your hospital resident representative about your coverage, and if none is available, contact your provincial or state medical association about available programs.

Buying Life Insurance

- Look for the lowest-cost renewable term insurance available.
- Do not be dazzled by the projections of "cash value" accumulations. These are usually based on assumptions favorable to the company.
- Whole life insurance is expensive and very rarely makes financial sense.
- Provincial and state medical association group plans may provide term insurance at one-half to one-fifth the cost of similar individual policies.
- Ask your association representative to comment on any deficiencies or agent claims existing in the group policy.
- Discuss your life insurance needs with the provincial or state medical association's insurance adviser to see what coverage (if any) you need. Many single physicians starting out in practice need none at all or just enough to cover their debts. Once they marry and have a family, their needs change. You should reassess your needs annually to cover any changes in your lifestyle.
- Even though they do not need any life insurance coverage, some physicians obtain the minimum unit amount from their local medical association to protect their future insurability. Failure to do so would jeopardize their ability to obtain future coverage if a medical problem develops.

Disability Insurance

Discuss your disability insurance needs with your provincial or state association's insurance adviser to determine whether you are adequately covered. You may be covered by the hospital for a portion of your income, but you might want to supplement this with an additional amount before starting out in practice. When you begin practice, estimate your expected income over the first 2 years and obtain the appropriate amount of disability coverage. As your income increases, your coverage can increase until it reaches the maximum allowed. Initially you may elect a low qualification period (e.g., 14 days) before receiving payments, but as your finances become more stable you can increase the length of this period and reduce the cost of premiums. Be sure to maximize benefits while you are healthy, as premiums and exclusions to coverage increase with any illness.

Compare your medical association's disability plan with those of private companies. You may find that some of these companies will not sell insurance coverage if you participate in your medical association's plan. Physicians who want more coverage than the association plan allows buy some coverage from a private company before buying more from the association. Before buying such a policy, however, ask your provincial or state association to review the private company's proposal. Your choice will depend on your annual earnings and the amount of protection you want. See the insurance agent of the medical association annually to reassess your needs.

Buying Disability Insurance

- Buy the insurance while you are healthy; you will not usually qualify after you become disabled!
- Check with your hospital representative to see whether you are already covered.
- You may want to supplement your present coverage through your medical association policy or a private plan.
- Medical association plans may be 30 to 60% cheaper than private plans.
- Be wary of agents' scare tactics and "smoke and mirror" tactics.
- Select a short "elimination period" until your finances are well established.
- Premiums are neither tax-deductible nor creditable, but benefits are not taxable.
- Ask your medical association's representative to comment on any deficiencies a private agent claims exist in the group policy.

Malpractice Insurance

In Canada, one body – the Canadian Medical Protective Association (CMPA), a mutual medical defense organization – provides professional liability protection to its members. CMPA coverage is mandatory. In the United States, details of malpractice coverage should be explored through state medical associations or the hospital or moonlighting establishment for which you are working.

Other Insurance

Risk management, automobile, health insurance after residency, and home-owner's insurance are further options to be explored with your broker.

OBTAINING A LOAN OR LINE OF CREDIT

- Banks are in business to make money from lending. They are not lending you money as a favor. Shop around! Residents are a great risk for banks. You should *not* be paying banking fees, annual fees, or credit card renewal fees!
- Be businesslike when dealing with your banker; see her by appointment and prepare complete and accurate documentation. You may want to suggest in the interview that you might want to do all your banking (personal and professional) at one branch if the deal is favorable.
- Ask for the prime rate on loans with variable interest rates. Make the banker justify any higher rate.
- A fair rate to expect is prime + ½ percent to prime + 1½ percent for a variable rate, but you may be able to negotiate better rates. A fixed rate is more expensive, but may be useful if you expect interest rates to rise.
- Establish a line of credit on which you can draw during the first 6 months so that you pay interest only on the funds you use.
- Through MD Management Limited, the Canadian Medical Association helps physicians who are setting up a practice to obtain loans at preferred rates through the National Bank. Other Canadian banks also try to woo professionals so shop around. Various US banks such as Citibank do so as well. Check with your union, housestaff association, or medical association representative for details and check out the websites below.
- You may wish to consolidate your students loans into a professional line of credit, thus securing a lower interest rate and allowing for tax deductions on interest charged.

Websites on Loans for Doctors

MedLending
   http://www.calumross.com/mortgages-for-physicians

Physician Loans
   www.physicianloans.com
National Association of Doctors
   www.nadonline.com
Life insurance rates
   www.term4sale.ca

HELP FROM OTHER PROFESSIONALS

Residents need help from other professionals, especially as they finish training and consider starting up a practice. Obtain references from your provincial or state medical association or from colleagues. The CIR also provides such information.

What a Good Accountant or Financial Planner Can Do for You

- Help you design/follow a monthly budget and help you strategize paying down your debt.
- Set up a record-keeping system for your practice when you start
- Provide you with monthly and formal financial statements that will summarize the financial health of your practice
- Help you budget and plan for the post-residency period
- Prepare income tax returns (some local medical associations offer income tax preparation services for residents at a reduced rate)
- Advise on financial investments
- Comment on the suitability of/timing for incorporating your practice
- Discuss retirement, estate, and tax planning

Choosing an Accountant

The ideal accountant should have the following:
- Experience with a medical practice
- Ability to communicate in a clear, concise, and professional manner
- Ability to provide responsible leadership for your financial affairs

Other Considerations

- Once the accountant sets up a bookkeeping system, make sure you have a good understanding of how it works.
- Ensure that the system is being maintained properly so that you are not paying the accountant for jobs that you could do yourself.
- Take your accountant with you when you consult with other financial advisers or grant permission for them to communicate. He or she will have a good understanding of your financial affairs and will be able to interpret any advice and its implications.

What a Good Lawyer Can Do for You

Ask the housestaff union for the name of the lawyer it retains to assist residents, usually free of charge, for matters related to residency (e.g., contract abuses). A good lawyer can also:

- Help you create a will (no matter how young you are!)
- Review contracts from employers (and help you to ensure that what was promised in a job interview is delivered contractually.[2]
- Draw up formal contracts between you and your co-workers when you start practice.
- Advise on lease agreements, mortgages, deeds, by-laws, and so on about the location of your practice.
- Advise on personal matters such as wills.
- Advise on investments, taxes, and so forth.
- Assist you in writing a will/living will.
- Create a trust or corporation to protect assets and reduce tax load.

Important Considerations in Dealing with a Lawyer

- Avoid choosing a friend as a business lawyer, as it may be awkward to change lawyers later.
- Ask your family lawyer, colleagues, or accountant to recommend a business lawyer.
- Ensure that the lawyer can communicate with you in a manner you can understand.
- Make the most of the time spent with the lawyer by making sure that your material is organized and that you are providing all the information he or she needs to do the job well.

What a Stockbroker Can Do for You

- Look after/buy-and-sell transactions
- Provide prompt, accurate execution of orders
- Provide a record of your holdings
- Make reliable market forecasts
- Provide timely technical and fundamental research
- Give insight into your investment needs

What a Real Estate Agent Can Do for You

- Connect you with a good mortgage broker
- Show you what is available for purchase and give expert appraisals
- Help you choose the best location for your office
- Help arrange details of leases
- Advise you on investment property
- Refer you to another agent on matters that are outside his area of expertise

What a Good Business Management Consultant Can Do for You

- Help you identify tax-credited educational investments for your children.
- Help set up a medical practice, including choosing a good location, training staff, and so on
- Offer expertise and problem solving on various aspects of the practice such as collections, income distribution, and partnership terms
- Help you prioritize financial costs (home purchase, debt payment, forming investment and credit strategies, etc.)
- Provide practice surveys and business analysis
- Give specialized consultation on financial investments, personal and family budgeting, and so forth

REFERENCES

1 *Guide to Establishing a Medical Practice.* MD Management Ltd, Ottawa (Much of this chapter is reprinted with permission from this guide.)
2 CMA Practice Management Curriculum for Medical Residents. 2015. At https://cma.ca/En/Pages/practice-management-curriculum.aspx

CHAPTER ELEVEN

I'm Finally Done: Now What?
Thoughts on the End of Residency

In Greek mythology, Procrustes was a robber who pretended to be an innkeeper on the road to Athens. Travelers seeking success in that city would stop at the inn, where Procrustes would tie them to a bed and adjust them to its length, cutting off the limbs of those who were too tall and stretching those who were too short. He was eventually killed by the hero Theseus.

Residency is truly a modern "Procrustean voyage," where conformity, even to deforming principles, can be the price of success. Musical, creative, playful, spontaneous, even romantic aspects of our lives may be cut off if we're not careful. There is no modern-day Theseus to intervene to preserve our integrity, to remind us of our need to remain whole. Our superiors and patients often expect too much of us.

Postgraduate medical education can be a time of great personal growth as well as stress and doubt. The completion of residency marks a departure from the many years of study and training and a shift toward independence and autonomy, away from attending physicians, senior residents, and the hospital hierarchy. Choices have to be made fairly with your partner and family about fellowships, subspecialties, private versus hospital practice, urban versus rural practice, and moves to new locations. Personal priorities have to be re-examined in the light of having more free time after years of living in an externally imposed structure. Debts wait unpaid. Residents sometimes feel emotionally numb at the end of their training, wondering if they will be able to maintain competence and empathy. They also experience mixed feelings of nostalgia or even loss over "moving on," and of pride and accomplishment, tinged with panic, in having become full-fledged physicians.

Various factors can make starting a practice a bit unnerving. Many patients have unrealistic expectations about their health and of their physicians, resulting in a marked increase in litigation against physicians. Malpractice claims in North America have more than doubled over the past 15 years. In Canada, patients may consult an excessive number of physicians because healthcare is perceived to be "free of charge." At the same time, provincial programs are being cut, hospitals closed, and the job mobility of new physicians curtailed. (Physician unemployment in some specialties has even been reported.) In the United States, many patients and some physicians have come to see their exchange as being based on profit and consumerism, and overseen by corporate insurance or managed-care companies that dictate policy and, indeed, what is to be considered acceptable treatment. In both countries constantly advancing technology emphasizes science over human experience and increasingly removes physicians from the bedside. Continuity of care and person-centeredness are lost. Overall, physicians find their decision-making power diminished or diluted. These developments and others, including slashed healthcare budgets, forced hospital mergers, and concerns about autonomy and wages, can significantly reduce job satisfaction for many.

For the last 20 years, the media has presented a worrying image of the physician–patient relationship. A large proportion of patients interviewed by *Time* magazine believed that physicians have no real interest in them; that only one in two "explains things well enough," and that physicians' prestige had declined over the previous 10 years.[1] *Time* concluded, "Never have doctors been able to do so much for their patients and rarely have patients seemed so ungrateful." New developments like "Dr Google," where patients make demands based on Internet research, up the ante of expectations even further. A survey conducted by the Association of American Medical Colleges[2] demonstrated that the majority of graduating medical students that year agreed that changes in the healthcare system had impaired physicians' independence. These students also believed that medicine would become less financially rewarding, that administrative and legal liabilities were increasingly burdensome, that a medical career interrupted family life too much, and that physicians will be even less respected over time. Finally – perhaps a final blow – a physician shortage is now evident in both the United States and Canada, particularly in rural and remote areas, and this implies a greater workload.[3]

Despite these trends, there are reasons to remain optimistic about the future of residency training and medicine in general in North America. New fields are flourishing, from psycho-immunology to genetic engineering to narrative medicine, new cures are pending, and there is an ever-growing emphasis on prevention. Exciting new technologies, like telemedicine, 3D printing and cyber-surgery links to underserviced communities, and an ever-expanding high-quality medical Internet are gaining new applications. A growing holistic movement with proponents such as Andrew Weil, MD, and Jon Kabat-Zinn, MD, have emphasized the mind–body connection, mindfulness, meditation, and how the physician–patient relationship has its own capacity to heal. Best of all, doctors are insisting on taking better care of themselves and are spending more time with their loved ones, and this makes them better physicians and happier, more resilient human beings.

OPTIONS AFTER RESIDENCY

The Fellowship and Research Option

Setting up practice is only one choice available to graduating residents. Other options include master's or doctorate degrees in medical ethics, research, business and management, health humanities, education, or public health epidemiology. Fellowships, which last from 1 to 3 years, fall into three categories: clinical, research, or combined.

A fellowship can provide an opportunity to develop a subspecialty, publish, and enhance the possibilities of an academic appointment. (In some university centers a fellowship, with resultant publications, is required before an academic appointment is granted.) It may allow you to sample a new university setting or city, postpone setting up practice, and clarify career plans. Discuss these issues with your mentor, residency director, or university fellowship officer. Matters to consider in negotiating a fellowship are similar to those in residency selection and include the following:

- Application procedures and interviewing
- Selection criteria (e.g., residency completion, provincial or state licensing) and degree of competition

- Benefits, funding, and salary (existence of a financial "ceiling" if one bills for patients seen)
- Office space and secretarial services
- Teaching, clinical, and call duties
- Publication expectations
- Assignment of credit or authorship for work done
- Possibility of grant renewal or ongoing funding
- Obligation to remain with the research department for a stipulated period on completion of the fellowship
- Availability or guarantee of a staff position after fellowship

Fellowship Funding

Many trainees begin doing research in medical school and residency and choose to continue after residency. The principal sources of fellowship funding in Canada are the Canadian Institutes of Health Research (CIHR), Health Canada, and the Natural Sciences and Engineering Research Council. Provincial funding is also available for specific projects, and the Royal College and College of Family Physicians in Canada also offer grants.

Current information on most fellowships available in the United States appears in the education issue that the *Journal of the American Medical Association* publishes every August (also available online). Information on federal research funding can be obtained from the National Institutes of Health, and Health Resources and Services Administration. Another resource is the American Physician and Scientist Association, at www.apsa.org. The number of subspecialty positions has actually been increasing in the United States over the past several years. *Index Medicus* has a listing of articles discussing pertinent topics relating to fellowships (administrative, pedagogical, and so on). It may be worthwhile doing a current-literature search on your area of interest. The AMA-FREIDA program also has a fellowship databank (see http://www.ama-assn.org/ama/pub/education-careers/graduate-medical-education/freida-online.page).

The fellowship office at the university at which you hope to train can provide information on deadlines, addresses, and the application procedures of provincial and state funding bodies. In addition, write to specialty associations, because they often offer funding or scholarships, and their databanks provide information on fellowships in North America. Other potential sources of funding include the following:

- Employment under attending physician ("staffman") grants
- Hospital research institutes
- Residency extension (postgraduate year 5 or 6)
- Junior staff appointments
- Philanthropic agencies such as the National Cancer Institute or Heart and Stroke Foundation
- Private industry (e.g., pharmaceutical companies)
- Self-funded clinical fellowships where one bills for patients seen
- Other foundation awards
- Scholarships/grants available through state, provincial, and national bodies

Academic Medicine

Many graduate specialists emerging from residency or fellowship training choose to embark on full-time university-based academic careers. Guidelines for selecting an academic position include clarifying:

- What academic rank will be offered in the position (e.g., lecturer vs assistant professor), and what mechanisms permit promotion
- Will you be assigned some other title (e.g., "Clinical Associate") and what are the advantages/disadvantages of this interim status?
- Whether tenure will be available and how it is granted
- Whether cross-appointments with other departments are permitted or encouraged
- What grants or financial resources are held by the department and how your income might be guaranteed
- Whether sabbaticals will be available and at what frequency
- What the mission statement of the medical school, hospital, department, and division are and whether these are compatible with your goals
- How much time will be allocated or protected for research versus clinical service
- Details of the research environment: lab personnel, office space, provision of materials and supplies (such as computer software)
- What support (e.g., mentoring/administrative) will be available for research start-up

- How much inpatient or outpatient clinical work is expected and what opportunities for teaching will be available
- Financial issues such as salaries, billing "ceilings" (and where surplus money goes when you surpass a ceiling), income split between salary and clinical work, benefits (insurance and leaves of absence), office selection and office staff, moving expense reimbursement
- Interview procedures (see chapter 2)

During final negotiations for the academic post, seek a written offer summarizing the above points. Discuss the offer with family, your spouse, friends, and possibly your lawyer, as they will all help you clarify ambiguities in the offer and uncertainties in your own mind.[4]

Locum Tenens

Many graduating residents feel unprepared to settle down in one practice or academic setting. They may wish to work part-time, travel, pay off student loans in a hurry, or explore cities where they might wish to settle eventually. The advantages of locum tenens (Latin for "place holder") positions include the large variety of practice settings, flexible scheduling, low office overhead, and low start-up fees and living expenses. You can find locums by word of mouth, through medical journals, licensing bodies, provincial or state medical association registries, or your professional specialty association. At least 25 medical placement agencies exist in the United States and Canada. See www.locumtenens.com and www.physicianwork.com. Visit your provincial or state medical association website for listings as well.

When negotiating with the placement agency or a specific medical facility, find out the mechanism of payment (hourly/daily, rates or fee for service), the overhead percentage deducted from your salary, and whether there is a minimum commitment time. Inquire whether you will be provided with provincial or state licensing, housing, and health and malpractice insurance. Don't be afraid to shop around or to negotiate firmly for benefits.

International, Humanitarian, and Volunteer Medicine

Many graduates decide to work part-time in a free, low-cost, or community-based clinic as a way of "giving something back" and enhancing skills for "hands-on, low technology" primary care. Most provinces and states can provide lists of public-health or community clinics. The Red Cross holds health fairs across the United States, and recruits volunteers for health screening programs. Other physicians seek experience abroad in Third World countries. Often contacts can be made through Canadian or American medical schools that have affiliate programs overseas or through agencies such as CUSO (Canadian Universities Services Overseas), the World Health Organization, and the Pan American Health Organization. Here are some specific resources for medical opportunities abroad:

- International Development Research Centre (http://www.idrc.ca/EN/Pages/default.aspx)
- Global Health Council (www.globalhealth.org)
- Health Volunteers Overseas (www.hvousa.org)
- International Federation of Medical Students' Associations (www.ifmsa.org)
- International Medical Corps (www.imcworldwide.org)
- Doctors of the World (http://doctorsoftheworld.org)
- Doctors Without Borders (www.msf.org)
- International Health Resource (www.amsa.org)
- Foreign and Commonwealth Office: Travel and living abroad (https://www.gov.uk/browse/abroad)
- Holt Medical Recruitment (http://www.holtmedical.com/workingabroad.htm)
- Masta Travelwell (http://www.masta-travel-health.com)
- Mediwork-Info (http://www.mediwork.info)
- Student Doc (http://www.studentdoctor.net)

Clinical Practice Options

Trying to decide where and how to set up a practice may prove daunting for the graduating resident. Options include group versus private versus hospital-based settings, salaried versus fee-for-service positions, HMOs, and public-versus private-sector institutions.

A new physician can join an already established group practice and pay overhead or buy into the partnership. Retiring physicians often sell their practices. See "Things to Consider," below.

Practice opportunities are usually listed in medical journals; on national, provincial, and state association websites; or sent to physicians by recruitment agencies ("head hunters"). Hiring a physician recruiter is one option. They work like a "head hunter" and can help you in three ways:[5]

1 They filter information and avoid a "web of confusion." They will do the legwork, field calls and inquiries, and match your preference and specifications to a potential employer.
2 They maximize exposure to an inner circle of hospitals and clinics that don't advertise and will be selective about whom they share your CV with.
3 They will take your working style, personal preferences, family needs, hobbies, and recreational interests into account and help you to select an appropriate job in an appropriate setting. They have links to realtors, chambers of commerce, etc.

Information on the geographical distribution of physicians in the United States can be found in an annual AMA publication *Physician Distribution and Medical Licenses* in the United States. The AMA also publishes a helpful, regularly updated guide entitled *Guide to Physician Success (GPS) Manual: A Guide for Young Physicians Transitioning from Residency into a Fellowship or Practice*.[6] Talk to your medical accountant about all options and financial and contractual obligations before signing on. Consider attending one of the AMA's annual practice management workshops for residents, which tour the country. Topics include "Starting Your Practice" and "Joining a Partnership or Group Practice." Information and up-to-date publications can be obtained from www.ama-assn.org.

In Canada, contact MD Management at www.mdm.ca regarding literature, practice workshops, and a list of financial advisers in your city or province familiar with these issues. Your specialty association website may have guidelines on entering practice as well. Another useful resource is www.drcareers.ca.

Things to Consider about Where and How You Want to Practice

• Family needs and preferences (job options for your spouse, schools for your children, community resources)

- Provincial/state licensing requirements restrictions (you'll need to apply for licensing and billing privileges at least nine months in advance of setting up practice)
- Type of practice:

  - Solo, group (single of multi-specialty)
  - Hospital- or university-based
  - Salaried or fee-for-service
  - Government/community clinics
  - HMO, PPO, or MSO (in the United States)

- Geography (city vs rural, weather, proximity to other families)
- Financial issues (cost of move, practice set-up, affordability of community re housing and cost of living)
- Contractual issues:

  - Salary, benefits, insurance coverage, bonuses, partnership options
  - Service, on-call and administrative responsibilities

- Collegiality, friendliness, and supportiveness of work setting
- Job satisfaction of physicians and support staff (i.e., a functional work setting!)
- Need for your clinical services/local competition levels (how long until your practice fills up?)
- Future prospects: can you grow in this job and this community?

Future Directions – A Note to Future Educators

Looking Back –

Learning to be a doctor arises out of a mixture of people, ideas, technical interventions, and experiences. Looking back at my time in psychiatry residency at the University of Illinois at Chicago, I am grateful for the times when I learned my physical and emotional limits and how to work up to and, at times, beyond them when needed. I am grateful for the well-rounded training in psychotherapy, psychopharmacology, leadership, and research. People who were kind enough to serve in the role of "patient" to my role of "doctor" still feel like they are with me, looking over my shoulder, or sometimes peering out from my heart.

The teachings of my mentors are still with me, in my heart and in my mind, shaping my commitment and calling to meet those who are suffering as fellow human beings. The hardest questions and issues are those that seem simple, but refuse to be answered simply, easily, or finally. Would I do it all again?

Difficult to say as I am still in the thick of it ...

SUMMARY

As you finish your residency, pat yourself on the back and celebrate with your loved ones, but remember that your learning does not stop there.[6] You will require continuing medical education as long as you call yourself a physician.[7] Give yourself permission to explore all your options: if you tire of clinical practice, you can conduct research, write, broadcast, consult, invent, administer, mediate, or become politically active around issues such as homelessness. You can work, teach, or consult in other countries. You can join academia and become the kind of professor who humanizes the experience of learning for both students and residents. Your vocation within medicine can change and grow as you do. Career counselling and medical executive coaching is now available to doctors to help them explore options. Doctors used to think they were "set for life" – now we realize we need to establish career goals on a regular basis, reinvent ourselves, and try new challenges just like any other professional.

Whatever your choice, remember the satisfaction of providing good and ethical care, of making accurate diagnoses, of helping someone feel better and regain a sense of dignity in the face of illness. Remember the honor of knowing what your patients have told you and no one else, and of being present at the key moments of their birth, life, and dying. Remember to thank your colleagues along the way. Always find that balance between lifestyle and service that our predecessors could not imagine or attain. As Sir William Osler reminds us:

> The practice of medicine is an art, not a trade; a calling, not a business; a calling in which your heart will be exercised equally with your head.

REFERENCES

1 Dolan B, Gwynne SC, Simpson JC. Sick and tired: Uneasy patients may be surprised to find their doctors are worried too. *Time*, 31 July 1989; 28–33. (More recently, a 2010 *Maclean's* magazine poll revealed that a growing number of Canadian patients don't trust their doctors. *Macleans*, 23 August 2010).

2 AAMC 2000 Graduate Questionnaire, cited in *New Physician*, May/June 2001; 4.

3 Cooper RA, Getzen TE, McKee HJ, et al. Economic and demographic trends signal an impending physician shortage. *Health Affairs* (Millwood). 2002;21(1):140–54. http://dx.doi.org/10.1377/hlthaff.21.1.140.

4 Pololi L. Career development for academic medicine – a nine step strategy. *BMJ Careers*. 2006;28(Jan):38–9.

5 Gresham R. The physician recruiter: Making your career transition a snap. At http://www.mommd.com/physicianrecruiters.shtml.

6 AMA. *Guide to Physician Success (GPS) Manual: A Guide for Young Physicians Transitioning from Residency into a Fellowship or Practice*. Chicago: 2009.

7 Edwards S, Puddester D. *Resident wellness and work/life balance in postgraduate medical education*. Future of Medical Education in Canada Postgraduate Project. 23

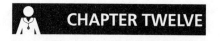

CHAPTER TWELVE

Knowledge Is Power: Social Media Guidelines

This chapter will review various sets of guidelines for the use of new technologies in learning and in communicating with colleagues and patients. The plea to use common sense rings loud and clear in all of them.

The use of social media has revolutionized our culture, including medicine and healthcare. A recent survey by MD Quantia found that 80% of physicians use social media for personal uses and 60 to 70% for professional purposes. Many doctors also interact with their patients or patients' family members, and 35% of them have received friend requests on platforms like Facebook from patients. Patients, because of their access to the Internet, become better informed around illness and treatment than they were before. This phenomenon has been called "Dr Google," and represents both a challenge and advantage to the care of patients.

TIP: "The Internet has democratized access to medical information. Just as it's easier for residents to look up information on any condition, it's easier for patients as well. It can be tempting to dismiss patients' own research, but they're often looking at the same sites we are. Finding out what patients have found online, talking about the specific information they found, and leading them toward other resources can often go a long way to assuaging patient fears and engaging patients in their own care."

The Federal State of Medical Boards (US), in its model policy guidelines for appropriate use of social media and social networks in medical practice, emphasizes that physicians must protect themselves from unintended consequences and should maintain the public's trust by protecting the confidentiality and privacy of their patients, avoiding requests for online medical advice, acting with professionalism, and being forthcoming about their employment, credentials, and potential conflicts of interest, and that they be aware that information they post online may become available to anyone and could be misconstrued. Indeed, patients often become curious about their healthcare providers, and seek access to information on their personal lives. This becomes relevant when residents, for example, use social media to date, network, log personal information, or post photos or other images. The guidelines suggest that doctors should be discouraged from interacting with patients on personal social networking platforms.

TIP: *"It is essential to keep accurate records of any communication with patients, just as one would write a note after any clinical encounter."*

Social networking websites can be useful places for doctors to gather and share their experiences, and to discuss diagnosis and treatment. It is recommended, however, that these networks be secured and password-protected. Patient privacy and confidentiality must be protected at all times. Information that could be used to identify a patient should never be included in electronic exchanges that might contravene privacy laws, such as HIPAA. Doctors who choose to write about patient encounters or their experiences as professionals must diligently disguise identifying data. When they post content online, they should remember that they are always representing the medical community and their standard of professionalism.

TIP: *"What has emerged over the past ten years is a semi-public sphere. In terms of disclosure, Facebook is somewhere between a phone call and the front page of a newspaper. But every electronic communication falls somewhere along that spectrum."*

TIP: "As a rule of thumb, don't email, text, or post online anything you wouldn't be comfortable seeing on the front page of a newspaper in an exposé of what residents say when they think nobody is looking."

To review their university and hospital institutions' policies on the use of social media, the Canadian Medical Association published a policy paper in 2011 called "Social Media and Canadian Physicians' Issues on Rules of Engagement." Their recommendations are provided here.

PATIENT CONFIDENTIALITY

- The privacy and security of individual patient information is paramount and should never be shared beyond the circle of care. This principle is also enshrined in CMA policy. In communicating with an individual patient in other than a face-to-face environment, a secure electronic communication platform must be used. Identifiable patient information, including images, should never be posted online or shared in electronic communications of a general nature.
- When using social media, physicians should endeavor to use the most stringent security and privacy settings available for the particular platform.

TIP: "In general, most email addresses are considered insecure. Most hospitals will grant residents a secure email address via which they can send identifying information about patients to other people with a secure address. Of course, information should only be sent if the recipient has a reason to receive it (e.g., it is being sent to another physician involved in that patient's care)."

- Physicians with employees should make them aware of issues concerning patient confidentiality in their own use of social media. Consideration should be given to instituting a social media policy for the office or practice.

- Social networking sites cannot guarantee confidentiality. Anything written on a social networking site can theoretically be accessed and made public. For example, the Patriot Act in the United States makes it possible for the US government under certain conditions to access any information posted on a social networking site or website hosted by a US service provider, even if this information is located within the "private or direct message" area of the site.

PROFESSIONALISM

- Having an online profile or identifiable presence on social media can have the same degree of positive or negative impact on a physician's social reputation as being active in any other public venue. In fact, having access to a global audience can magnify this reputation.
- The most effective use of social media often involves communicating information that is both personal and professional. However, physicians must retain the appropriate boundaries of the patient–physician relationship when dealing with individual patients. The same standards of professionalism that would apply in face-to-face physician–patient interactions also apply in electronic interactions.

TIP: "It's annoying to perform a patient assessment or a complicated procedure only to be paged midway through. Many residents now text each other where once they might have paged. Texting has advantages over paging: it's asynchronous, which means that residents can respond at their leisure, and one can put a lot more information into a text message than into a short pager callback number."

- If a physician is an employee of a healthcare institution or organization that has social media guidelines in place, he or she should review these and act accordingly.

ONLINE COMMUNICATION ISSUES

- Electronic communications are not anonymous and are always stored in some form. As such, it is possible to trace the author of a comment even if posted anonymously.

- Once their material is published online, authors of comments on social media sites no longer control how and where the information is disseminated, and these comments can sometimes lose context.

TIP: *"Patients may sometimes want to communicate electronically. Requests for this will only increase. After all, virtually every other profession now conducts large amounts of business online. E.g., If you are going to communicate with patients via email, it is often helpful to get a signed consent and document that you've discussed the risks and benefits with the patient, as with any medical procedure. Again, it can be helpful to contact the privacy officer at your hospital, as many hospitals have policies around electronic communication with patients and may even have standard consent forms for physicians and patients to sign."*

- Postings to social media sites are subject to the same laws of how patients and members of the public seek information about health and increase the sense of engagement patients have in their own care. Through a variety of websites and fuelled by the growing availability of electronic patient health records, patients are increasingly sharing information with other patients about their health conditions and their healthcare providers.

THE NEW MEDIA, PROFESSIONALISM, AND CONFIDENTIALITY

The rapidity with which we can share information about ourselves and others is a mixed blessing. Here are some tips for avoiding professional breeches.

Digital Professionalism Framework

1 Keep your profile accurate and up to date: some will take your profile as the literal truth, others will be intrinsically skeptical. Maintaining a principle of honesty, even if playful, is important in dealing with reinterpretation and misinterpretation. Principle #1: Establish and sustain an online professional

presence that befits your responsibilities while representing your interests ... but be selective where you establish a profile.

2 Manage access to different parts of your profile: professional dimensions more public and personal dimensions more private. Without the ability to manage different parts of your life they will tend to blur together, with possibly serious consequences. Principle #2: Use privacy controls to manage more personal parts of your online profile and do not make public anything that you would not be comfortable defending as professionally appropriate in a court of law.

3 Reflect on how your actions will be perceived by others: The appropriateness and perception of online postings can be very hard to judge without taking a clear, conscientious approach to writing and posting online. Principle #3: Think carefully and critically about how what you say or do will be perceived by others, and act with appropriate restraint.

4 Your actions will reflect on your profession and institution: an act appropriate in one context may not be in another, particularly if an individual is linked to a profession or institution. The actions of the individual can be seen as reflecting or criticizing the position of the institution, even if not intended. Principle #4: Think carefully and critically about how what you say or do reflects on others, both individuals and organizations, and act with appropriate restraint.

5 Deal with ambient and permanent surveillance: Almost everything you do online can be monitored and recorded (e.g., Google searches, Facebook postings). Comments and postings may be visible years later and could affect an individual's ability to get or retain a job. Principle #5: Think carefully and critically about how what you say or do will be perceived in years to come; consider every action online as permanent.

6 Deal with hostile acts: individuals may seek to tarnish or even destroy another's reputation online (postings, ratings) or impersonate them (identity theft). Principle #6: Be aware of the potential for attack or impersonation; know how to protect

your online reputation and what steps to take when it is under attack.

7 Work responsibly and positively within online communities: although there may not be the same explicit duties of service and care within an online community, the professional's role within society should extend to the virtual as well as to the real. Principle #7: An online community is still a community and you are still a professional there.

8 Honesty and accountability: impersonation and deception are easy to achieve in online environments, but that doesn't make them appropriate. Principle #8: Pretence and deceit are inappropriate behaviors for health professionals. Do not impersonate another or seek to hide your identity in any professional interaction unless professionally required, as in an anonymous peer review.

9 Criminal behavior: just because it's online doesn't mean it's free or available for you to do what you want with it. Principle #9: Theft and piracy are not acceptable forms of behavior for any professionals (accept perhaps for gangsters). Work within the law.

10 Standards: respect and openness are not optional, even if you're just using email or texting. Principle #10: Behave professionally and respectfully in all venues and using all media.

Used with permission: Ellaway R and Tworek J (2012), The net generation illusion: Challenging conformance to social expectations. In Ferris SP, *Teaching, Learning and the Net Generation: Concepts and Tools for Reaching Digital Learners*. Developed from an earlier version in Ellaway R, eMedical teacher: Digital professionalism, *Medical Teacher* 2010;32(8):705–7

TIP: *"As a matter of politeness, I refrain from checking my smartphone for anything in front of a patient. I treat my smartphone like I treat my pager, like I treat any bodily function: It's best done outside the patient's room, ideally in private."*

DRIVING THE POINT HOME, AGAIN! – SOCIAL NETWORKING DOS AND DON'TS

Follow these six tips provided by AMSA to safeguard your professional reputation and protect your medical career from being tarnished (or even destroyed):

1 *Privacy is critical.* Stifle the urge to tell the world about that extremely rare and fascinating case you experienced that day. Remember that information can potentially identify a patient, even without divulging a patient's name or social security number. Safeguarding protected health information is not only an ethical obligation, but a legal one.
  Check your school's policy. Whether your school has a specific policy on online conduct or a general code of professionalism, you may be forced to interpret what is appropriate versus inappropriate. Use good judgment and always avoid criticizing your school, professors, and deans online.

2 *Think before your write.* Consider everything that you write on the internet as permanent – there is no undo online. While you may be able to delete a post or comment, it is usually archived somewhere and accessible in the future. Quick reference: if you would be embarrassed if your Dean read your statements, then you're better off not posting them.

3 *Clean up your Facebook page.* Don't use a profile picture of you holding a bottle of Jack Daniels from your friend's last party. Physician recruiters and residency programs regularly check Facebook to screen and identify candidates. Use the privacy settings with Facebook, but remember that such controls are only a deterrent, not an absolute insulator. In addition, exercise your right to un-tag yourself from photos or ask your friends to take compromising photos down.

4 *Not so funny.* What you think is funny may be considered inappropriate and offensive by others. Try to limit the use of jokes on social network sites unless you think it's clean and funny enough that your future employer might laugh.

5 *Pick your friends carefully.* Consider wisely before adding patients as "friends" on Facebook or other social networks. And if your friends post questionable information on your Facebook wall, delete it immediately.

Source: AMSA, *The New Physician* (by Paul Wynn)

CHAPTER THIRTEEN

Helpful Resources and Recommended Reading

Websites, other resources, and suggested readings for each chapter follow. This format will allow you to learn more about specific themes, challenges, opportunities, resources, and strategies covered in each chapter.

CHAPTER ONE

Recommended Reading

Edmonstone J. *Personal Resilience for Healthcare Staff: When the Going Gets Tough*. London: Radcliffe Publishing Ltd; 2013.

Jauhar S. *Doctored: The Disillusionment of an American Physician*. New York: Farrar, Straus and Giroux; 2014.

Kopacz DR. *Re-Humanizing Medicine: A Holistic Framework for Transforming Your Self, Your Practice, and the Culture of Medicine*. Washington: Ayni Books; 2014.

CHAPTER TWO

Applying for Residency and Tips on the Match

AMA-FREIDA (Fellowship and Residency Electronic Interactive Database). Computer listing of residencies. Access with data on programs and institutions. American Medical Association and Resident Physician Section (AMA-RPA). Check out the "Resources

for Residents" section of the AMA website (ama-assn.org) for regularly updated content on navigating the match, transitioning in residency, contract information, preparing a CV, resident work-hours policies, and student-loan debt relief.
www.ama-assn.org

AMA Directory of Graduate Medical Education Programs (published yearly)

AMA Medical Student Section
http://amaMedStudent.org

American Academy of Family Physicians
www.aafp.org/online/en/home.html

AAFP. Directory of Family Medicine Residency Programs
http://www.aafp.org/residencies

AAFP. *Strolling through the Match*
http://www.aafp.org/medical-school-residency/residency/match.html?cmpid=_van_711

AAFP. Virtual Family Medicine Interest group. Covers issues related to research, choosing a residency, arranging interviews, navigating the match, and relocating.
http://www.aafp.org/medical-school-residency.html

American Association of Medical Colleges. Council of Teaching Hospitals Directory (published yearly)

American College of Physicians Residency Search Database
www.acponline.org/residency/index.html

American Medical Students' Association. AMSA Online Residency Directory
www.amsa.org

Canadian Resident Matching Service
www.carms.ca

Educational Commission for Foreign Medical Graduates
www.ecfmg.org

Electronic Residency Application Service (ERAS)
www.aamc.org/students/eras

Find a Resident
www.aamc.org/students/findaresident

Interactive Internal Medicine Residency Database
http://www.acponline.org/medical_students/residency/find

National Residency Matching Program (USA), Data and Reports.
http://www.nrmp.org/match-data/main-residency-match-data

Residency 101.com
http://www.residencyandfellowship.com/Main_Page

Resident Career Counseling
www.acponline.org/counseling

Strolling Through the Match
www.aafp.org/strolling

The Successful Match
www.MD2B.net

Recommended Reading

AMSA's Student Guide to Appraisal and Selection of Housestaff Training Programs. AMSA, Reston, VA; see www.amsa.org.

Annual Report on Graduate Medical Education (yearly in December issue of *JAMA*).

Association of American Medical Colleges. *Roadmap to Residency: Understanding the Process of Getting into Residency.* 2015 ed. www.aamc.org/roadmaptoresidency

Freedman J. *The Residency Interview: How to Make the Best Possible Impression.* New York: MedEdits Publishing; 2010.

Freeman B. *The Ultimate Guide to Choosing a Medical Speciality.* 3rd ed. New York: McGraw-Hill Medical; 2012.

Iserson KV. *Iserson's Getting into a Residency: A Guide for Medical Students.* Tucson: Galen Press; 2013.

Katta R, Desai S. *The Successful Match: 200 Rules to Succeed in the Residency Match.* Houston: Md2b; 2009.

Peterkin A. There are some questions residency interviewers have no right to ask. *Can Med Assoc J.* 1989;140:325

Taylor A. *How to Choose a Medical Specialty,* 4th ed. Philadelphia: Saunders; 2003

CHAPTER FOUR

Residents' Organizations

Canada

Resident Doctors of Canada (RDoc), formerly Canadian Association of Internes and Residents
http://residentdoctors.ca

Canadian Federation of Medical Students
http://www.cfms.org/index.php?lang=en

British Columbia: The Professional Association of Residents of British Columbia (PAR-BC)
www.par-bc.org

Alberta: The Professional Association of Resident Physicians of Alberta (PARA)
www.para-ab.ca

Saskatchewan: The Professional Association of Internes and Residents of Saskatchewan (PAIRS)
http://www.saskresidents.ca

Manitoba: The Professional Association of Residents and Interns of Manitoba (PARIM)
www.parim.org

Ontario: The Professional Association of Internes and Residents of Ontario (PAIRO)
www.pairo.org

Quebec: Fédération des Médecins Résidents du Québec (FMRQ)
www.fmrq.qc.ca

Maritimes (Nova Scotia, New Brunswick, and Prince Edward Island): The Professional Association of Residents in the Maritime Provinces (PARI-MP)
www.parimp.ca

Newfoundland/Labrador: The Professional Association of Internes and Residents of Newfoundland (PAIRN)
http://www.pairn.ca/home.aspx

United States

American Medical Association – Resident and Fellow Section
http://www.ama-assn.org/ama/pub/about-ama/our-people/
member-groups-sections/resident-fellow-section.page

CIR (Committee of Interns and Residents)
www.cirseiu.org

CIR Florida
305–325–8922

CIR Massachusetts
617–414–5301

CIR New Mexico
505–508–3306

CIR New York/New Jersey
info@cirseiu.org

CIR Northern California
510–464–8011

CIR Southern California
310–329–0111

CIR Washington, DC
202–872–5838

United Kingdom

British Medical Association Junior Doctors
http://bma.org.uk

The Doctor's Coach
www.thedoctorscoach.co.uk

Wellness Resources

American Academy of Family Practitioners
http://www.aafp.org/home.html

AAFP, Balancing Act Series:

Compassion Fatigue: http://www.aafp.org/fpm/2000/0400/p39.html
The Day Care Stare: http://www.aafp.org/fpm/2003/1000/p80.html
The 80/20 Rule of Time Management: http://www.aafp.org/
fpm/2000/0900/p76.html
15 Tips for Managing Life at Work and Home: http://www.aafp.
org/fpm/2000/0200/p60.html
5 Priority Setting Traps: www.aafp.org/fpm/20010400/60five.html
5 Ways to Say No Effectively: www.aafp.org/fpm/980700fm/
balance.html
Grieving the Death of a Patient: www.aafp.org/
fpm/20000500/78grie.html
Ideas for Managing Stress and Extinguishing Burnout: www.aafp.
org/fpm/20020400/35eigh.html
Life Balance: 17 Tips from Doctors for Doctors: www.aafp.org/
fpm/20010600/60life.html
Preventing Burnout: www.aafp.org/fpm/20000400/70prev.html
Running on Empty: www.aafp.org/fpm/20000100/68runn.html
6 Ways to Make Play a Priority: www.aafp.org/fpm/990100fm/
balancing.html

American Medical Student Association, Medical Student Well-Being
http://www.amsa.org/AMSA/Homepage/About/Committees/
WellBeing.aspx

Association of Gay and Lesbian Psychiatrists
www.aglp.org

CAIR Position Paper on Resident Well-being
http://residentdoctors.ca

Canadian Association of Physicians with Disabilities
www.capd.ca

Canadian Medical Association's Med Student Centre
https://www.cma.ca/En/Pages/medical-students.aspx

CMA Guide to Physician Health and Well-being
https://www.cma.ca/Assets/assets-library/document/en/
advocacy/policy-research/CMA_Policy_Physician_health_and_well-
being_PD98-04-e.pdf

Center for Professional Health
www.mc.vanderbilt.edu/root/vumc.php?site=cph

Doctors' Health Matters: Finding the Balance
www/cma.ca_Health_and_Wellbeing/physician_health_conference/
PHWB-2008conf-report_e.pdf

ePhysicianhealth.com
eWorkplacehealth.com

Foundation for Medical Excellence
www.tfme.org

Gay and Lesbian Medical Association
www.glma.org

Healthy Living (Heart and Stroke Foundation Canada)
www.heartandstroke.com

Physical Activity Guides
http://www.hc-sc.gc.ca/hl-vs/physactiv/index-eng.php

Resident Doctors of Canada
http://residentdoctors.ca

Stress Management for Physicians
www.texmed.org/Template.aspx?id=4619

Physician Health

Canada

Canadian Federation of Medical Students
www.cfms.org

Canadian Medical Foundation
http://medicalfoundation.ca

Canadian Physicians' Health Network
https://www.cma.ca/index.cfm/ci_id/25567/la_id/1.htm

Fédération des médecins résidents du Québec
www.fmrq.qc.ca

Federation of Medical Women in Canada
http://fmwc.ca

Resident Doctors of Canada
http://residentdoctors.ca

University of Ottawa Faculty Wellness Program
www.medicine.uottawa.ca/wellness

University of Toronto Resident Wellness
http://www.pgme.utoronto.ca/content/resident-wellness

United States

American Foundation for Suicide Prevention
www.afsp.org

Federation of State Physicians Health Programs
www.fsphp.org

International

International Alliance for Physician Health
http://physicianhealth.ning.com

Other Resources

Film

Carpe Diem (available online at ePhysicianHealth.com and
Youtube.com)

Podcasts

Healthy Practices: https://www.cma.ca/physicianhealth

Discussion Groups

CMA Healthy Practices group: www.asklepios.ca

Recommended Reading

AFMC Resource Group on Physician Health and Well-being:
Report to the AFMC Board of Directors, May 2010. Updates
available.

Bolton G. *Reflective Practice: Writing and Professional Development.* 4th
ed. Los Angeles: Sage Publications; 2014.

Brady, DW. What's important to you? The use of narratives to promote selfreflection and to understand the experiences of medical residents. *Ann Int Med.* 2002;137:220–3.

Cole T, Goodrich TJ, Gritz E (eds). *Faculty Health in Academic Medicine.* New York: Humana Press; 2009.

Gautam, M. *Iron Doc: Practical Stress Management Tools for Physicians.* Ottawa: Self-published; 2004.

Gautam M, ed. *CanMEDS Physician Health Guide: A Practical Handbook for Physician Health and Wellbeing.* Ottawa: Royal College of Physicians and Surgeons of Canada; 2009.

Goldman L, Myers M, Dickstein L. *The Handbook for Physician Health: The Essential Guide to Understanding the Health Care Needs of Physicians.* Chicago: American Medical Association; 2000.

Handler C, Handler C, Gill D. *English and Reflective Writing Skills in Medicine: A Guide for Medical Students and Doctors.* London: Radcliffe Medical Press; 2011.

Kahn N Jr, Schaeffer H. A process group approach to stress reduction and personal growth in a family practice residency program. *J Fam Pract.* 1981;12:1043–7.

Lipsenthal L. *Finding Balance in a Medical Life: A Guided Program to Help You Reclaim a Sense of Balance in Your Busy Life in Medicine.* Lee Lipsenthal; 2007.

Matthews DA, Classen DC, Willms JL. A program to help interns cope with stresses in an internal medicine residency. *J Med Educ.* 1988;63:539–47.

Rabow MW. Doctoring to heal: Fostering well-being among physicians through personal reflection. *West J Med.* 2001;174:66–9.

Remen RN. Recapturing the soul of medicine: Physicians need to reclaim meaning in their working lives. *West J Med.* 2001;174:4–5.

Scott CD, Hawk J (eds). *Heal Thyself: The Health of Health Care Professionals.* New York: Brunner/Mazel; 1986.

Sotile WM, Sotile MO. *The Resilient Physician: Effective Emotional Management for Doctors and Their Medical Organizations.* Washington: American Medical Association; 2002.

Southwick SM, Charney DS. *Resilience: The Science of Mastering Life's Greatest Challenges.* Cambridge: Cambridge University Press; 2012. http://dx.doi.org/10.1017/CBO9781139013857.

Spiegel J. *The Mindful Medical Student: A Psychiatrist's Guide to Staying Who You Are While Becoming Who You Want to Be.* Hanover: Dartmouth College Press; 2009.

Straus S, Sackett D. *Mentorship in Academic Medicine*. London: BMJ
Books; 2013. http://dx.doi.org/10.1002/9781118446065.

Wicks RJ. *Overcoming Secondary Stress in Medical and Nursing Practice:
A Guide to Professional Resilience and Personal Well-being*. New York:
Oxford University Press; 2005.

CHAPTER FIVE

Centre for Interprofessional Education
www.ipe.utoronto.ca

Useful Networking Sites for Residents

https://www.aamc.org/cim/residency/programs/
(Residency section)

www.amsa.org (see Resident section, including the journal *New
Physician*)

www.ama-assn.org/ama/pub/about-ama/our-people/member-
groups-sections/resident-fellow-section/rfs-resources/residency-
vacancies-work-environment/find-residency-fellowship.page

www.healthcommunities.com

www.ResidencyandFellowship.com

www.residentphysician.com

www.residentweb.com

www.scutwork.com

Recommended Reading

Gawande A. What Doctors Don't Learn about Death and Dying.
TED talk. http://ideas.ted.com/death-and-the-missing-piece-of-
medical-school/.

Guerrasio J. *Remediation of the Struggling Medical Learner*. Irwin, PA:
Association for Hospital Medical Education; 2013.

Nelson S, Tassone M, Hodges B. *Creating the Health Care Team of the
Future: The Toronto Model for Interprofessional Education and Practice*.
Ithaca, NY: ILR Press; 2014.

Thistlethwaite JE. *Values-based Interprofessional Collaborative Practice: Working Together in Health Care*. Cambridge: Cambridge University Press; 2012. http://dx.doi.org/10.1017/CBO9781139108904.

CHAPTER SIX

Resources for Physician Health and Help with Substance Abuse

American Society of Addiction Medicine
www.asam.org

Canadian Physician Health Institute
http://cphi-icsm.ca/

Federation of State Physician Health Programs
www.fsphp.org

Ontario Medical Association Physician Health Program
https://www.oma.org/Pages/default.aspx

Substance Abuse and Mental Health Services Administration
www.samhsa.gov

Talbott Recovery Campus
www.talbottcampus.com

Medical Spouses

AMA Alliance
www.amaalliance.org

American College of Osteopathic Family Physicians
http://www.acofp.org/

Auxiliary to the National Medical Association
http://www.anmanet.org/

International Medical Spouse Network
www.medicalspouse.org

Southern Medical Association Alliance
http://sma.org/

Cultural Competency

Center for Cross Cultural Health
410 Church St., Suite W227, Minneapolis, MN, 55455

Cross Cultural Health Care Program
http://xculture.org

Interface International
3821 East State St., Suite 197, Rockford, IL, 61108

Office of Minority Health (USA)
http://minorityhealth.hhs.gov

United States Department of Health and Human Services
http://www.hhs.gov/

Recommended Reading

Bailey RK. *A Doctor's Prescription for Health Care Reform: The National Medical Association Tackles Disparities, Stigma, and the Status Quo.* Bloomington: Westbow Press; 2013.

Barr DA. *Health Disparities in the United States: Social Class, Race, Ethnicity, and Health.* 2nd ed. Baltimore: Johns Hopkins University Press; 2014.

Bigby JA, ed. *Cross-Cultural Medicine.* Philadelphia: American College of Physicians; 2003.

Bleakley A. *Patient-centred Medicine in Transition: The Heart of the Matter.* Cham: Springer; 2014. http://dx.doi.org/10.1007/978-3-319-02487-5.

Boorman S. *NHS Health and Well-Being Review: Final Report.* London: Department of Health; 2010.

Colgan R. *Advice to the Healer: On the Art of Caring.* 2nd ed. New York: Springer; 2013. http://dx.doi.org/10.1007/978-1-4614-5170-9.

Collins JC, Rocco TS, Bryant LO, eds. *Health and Wellness Concerns for Racial, Ethnic, and Sexual Minorities: New Directions for Adult and Continuing Education.* San Francisco: Jossey-Bass; 2014.

Donhoe M, ed. *Public Health and Social Justice.* San Francisco: Jossey-Bass; 2012.

Dreachslin JL, Gilbert MJ, Malone B. *Diversity and Cultural Competence in Health Care: A Systems Approach.* San Francisco: Jossey-Bass; 2012.

Harvey VL, Hounsel TH. *Health Care Disparities and the LGBT Population*. Lanham: Lexington Books; 2014.

Hurwitz B, Sheikh A, eds. *Health Care Errors and Patient Safety*. London: BMJ Books; 2009.

Klass P. *Treatment Kind and Fair: Letters to a Young Doctor*. New York: Basic Books; 2008.

Koenig HG. *Spirituality in Patient Care: Why, How, When, and What*. 3rd ed. West Conshohocken: Templeton Press; 2013.

Mayo Clinic Center for Social Media. *Bringing the Social Media Revolution to Health Care*. Mayo Foundation for Medical Education & Research; 2012.

McLean CL, ed. *Creative Arts in Human Medicine*. Edmonton: Brush Education; 2014.

Ofri D. *What Doctors Feel: How Emotions Affect the Practice of Medicine*. Boston: Beacon Press; 2013.

Perez MA, Luquis RR. *Cultural Competence in Health Education and Health Promotion*. 2nd ed. San Francisco: Jossey-Bass; 2013.

Pizzorno JE, Murray MT. *Textbook of Natural Medicine*. 4th ed. London: Churchill Livingstone; 2012.

Pukall CF. *Human Sexuality: A Contemporary Introduction*. Toronto: Oxford University Press; 2014.

Purnell LD, Paulanka BJ. *Transculutral Health Care: A Culturally Competent Approach*. 2nd ed. Philadelphia: FA Davis; 2003.

Ruger JP. *Health and Social Justice*. Oxford: Oxford University Press; 2012.

Sanders L. *Every Patient Tells a Story: Medical Mysteries and the Art of Diagnosis*. Easton, PA: Harmony; 2010.

Selzer R. *Letters to a Young Doctor*. New York: Mariner Books; 2013.

Shoenberg P, Yakeley J, eds. *Learning about Emotions in Illness: Integrating Psychotherapeutic Teaching into Medical Education*. New York: Routledge; 2014.

Silverman J, Kurtz S, Draper J. *Skills for Communicating with Patients*. 3rd ed. London: Radcliffe Medical Press; 2013.

Smith C. *How to Succeed at the Medical Interview*. 2nd ed. London: BMJ Books; 2013. http://dx.doi.org/10.1002/9781118393796.

Spector RE. *Cultural Diversity in Health and Illness*. 8th ed. Upper Saddle River, NJ: Prentice Hall; 2012.

Stewart M, et al. *Patient-centered Medicine: Transforming the Clinical Method*. 3rd ed. Abingdon: Radcliffe Medical Press; 2014.

Storti C. *Cross-Cultural Dialogues: 74 Brief Encounters with Cultural Differences*. Yarmouth, MA: Intercultural Press; 1994.

Topol E. *The Patient Will See You Now: The Future of Medicine Is in Your Hands*. New York: Basic Books; 2015.

Truog RD, Browning DM, Johnson JA. *Talking with Patients and Families about Medical Error: A Guide for Education and Practice*. Baltimore: Johns Hopkins University Press; 2011.

Wachter R. *Understanding Patient Safety*. 2nd ed. New York: McGraw-Hill Professional; 2012.

Wylie KR, editor. *ABC of Sexual Health*. 3rd ed. London: BMJ Books; 2015.

CHAPTER SEVEN

Accreditation Council for Medical Education
www.acgme.org

Educational Commission for Foreign Medical Graduates
www.ecfmg.org

Electronic Residency Application Support for IMGs
www.ecfmg.org/eras

Foundation for Advancement of International Medical Education
www.faimer.org

International Federation of Medical Students
www.ifmsa.org

Recommended Reading

Alguire PC, Whelan GP, Rajput V. *The International Medical Graduate's Guide to US Medicine and Residency Training*. Philadelphia: American College of Physicians; 2008.

Bowman MA, Frank E, Allen DI. *Women in Medicine: Career and Life Management*. 3rd ed. New York: Springer; 2011.

Braude HD. *Intuition in Medicine: A Philosophical Defense of Clinical Reasoning*. Chicago: University of Chicago Press; 2012. http://dx.doi.org/10.7208/chicago/9780226071688.001.0001.

Ewseudo R. *Medical Speciality Training in the United States of America: A Must Have Roadmap for International Medical Graduates.* Denver: Outskirts Press; 2012.

Femgren GB. *Medicine and Religion: A Historical Introduction.* Baltimore: Johns Hopkins University Press; 2014.

Figley CR, Huggard P, Rees CE. *First Do No Self-Harm: Understanding and Promoting Physician Stress Resilience.* New York: Oxford, 2013. http://dx.doi.org/10.1093/acprof:oso/9780195383263.001.0001.

Harvey VL, Hounsel TH. *Health Care Disparities and the LGBT Population.* Lanham: Lexington Books; 2014.

Koenig HG. *Spirituality in Patient Care: Why, How, When, and What.* 3rd ed. West Conshohocken: Templeton Press; 2013.

Math K. *Surviving Residency: A Medical Spouse Guide to Embracing the Training Years.* 2nd ed., C and B Press; 2013.

Sandberg S. *Lean In: Women, Work, and the Will to Lead.* New York: Knopf; 2013.

Wylie KR, editor. *ABC of Sexual Health.* 3rd ed. London: BMJ Books; 2015.

CHAPTER EIGHT

Exam Preparation

National Board of Medical Examiners Web-Based Self-Assessment Services
www.nbme.org/sas

Journals of Medical Education

Academic Medicine
http://journals.lww.com/academicmedicine/

Advances in Health Sciences Education
www.springer.com

BMC Medical Education
www.biomedcentral.com/bmcmededuc/

Journal of Continuing Education in the Health Professions
http://onlinelibrary.wiley.com/journal/10.1002/%28ISSN%291554-558X

Journal of the International Association of Medical Science Educators
www.iamse.org

Medical Teacher
www.medicalteacher.org

Teaching and Learning in Medicine
http://www.tandfonline.com/toc/htlm20/current#.VQb8NI7F9qU

CME Websites

AMA-CME Select
http://www.ama-assn.org/ama/pub/education-careers/continuing-medical-education.page

American College of Physicians Journal Club
https://acpjc.acponline.org/

American Medical Association. Medical science and education
www.ama-assn.org/ama/pub/category/2797.html
http://www.ama-assn.org/ama/pub/physician-resources/medical-science.page

Canadian Medical Association. CME online
https://www.cma.ca/En/Pages/continuing-medical-education.aspx

CME Calendar
https://iicme.com

CME Gateway
http://www.cmegateway.org

CME Web
www.cmeweb.com/gindex.php

Doctor's Guide to Medical Conferences and Meetings
http://www.docguide.com/crc

Health on the Net: Conferences and Events
www.hon.ch/cgi-bin/conferences

Journal of Family Practice Journal Club
http://www.jfponline.com

Stanford primary care teaching modules
ctm.stanford.edu

Search Tools for Medical Information

Health on the Net Foundation
www.hon.ch

Medical Matrix
www.medmatrix.org
http://medmatrix.org/index.asp

Medical World Search
www.mwsearch.com/mwsframetemplate.htm?

Medscape
www.Medscape.com

Useful Medical Websites

American Hospital Directory
www.ahd.com

American Medical Association
www.ama-assn.org

Canadian Medical Association Online
www.cma.ca

College of Family Physicians of Canada
www.cfpc.ca

Medical Matrix. More than 2000 links with annotated sites
www.medmatrix.org

U.S. National Library of Medicine
www.nlm.nih.gov

Databases

Agency for Healthcare Research and Quality
www.ahrq.gov

Cochrane Database of Systematic Reviews (COCH)
Includes full text of regularly updated systematic reviews of healthcare prepared by the Cochrane Collaboration
www.cochrane.org

Current Contents. References of 7500 journals. Pay per use. Efficient gateway to psychiatric periodicals via its medical link
http://ip-science.thomsonreuters.com/index.html

Medline. A pillar of medical research databases that you can access a number of ways
https://www.nlm.nih.gov/bsd/pmresources.html

Medweb electronic newsletters and journals
www.healthlibrary.emory.edu

PubMed
http://www.ncbi.nlm.nih.gov/pubmed

Society of Teachers of Family Medicine
http://www.stfm.org

Virtual Hospital
http://www.uiowa.edu/health-care

Virtual Medical Library / Cliniweb
http://www.ohsu.edu/xd

Medical Journal Internet Addresses

Ask your program / hospital librarian / specialty association how to obtain free access to online journals in your field.

Medical Literature Websites

Cochrane Library
www.cochrane.org

Medline by Pub Med
www.ncbi.nlm.nih.gov/sites/entrez

York Systematic Reviews
www.crd.york.ac.uk/crdweb

Online Journal Clubs

ACP Journal Club
https://acpjc.acponline.org

Bandolier
http://www.medicine.ox.ac.uk/bandolier

CFPC Critical Appraisal
http://www.cfp.ca/site/misc/cfp_interactive.xhtml

Essential Evidence Plus
http://www.essentialevidenceplus.com

Info Poems: Journal of Family Practice
http://www.jfponline.com

Clinical Practice Guidelines

National Guidelines Clearinghouse
www.guideline.gov

Primary Care Clinical Practice Guidelines
http://medicine.ucsf.edu/education/resed/ebm/practice_
guidelines.html

Specialty Board Exams

Canada

Medical Council of Canada
www.mcc.ca

Royal College of Physicians and Surgeons of Canada
www.rcpsc.medical.org
http://www.royalcollege.ca/portal/page/portal/rc/public

United States

Federation of State Medical Boards
www.fsmb.org

National Board of Medical Examiners
www.nbme.org

United States Medical Licensing Examination
www.usmle.org

Resident Researchers/PhD Students

Centre for Learning in Practice
www.rcpsc.medical.org/clip/

NIH Medical Scientist Training Program
http://www.nigms.nih.gov/Training/InstPredoc/Pages/
PredocOverview-MSTP.aspx

Society for Humanists and Social Scientists and Medicine / American
Physician Scientists Association
http://scholarsinmedicine.blogspot.ca

US Department of Health and Human Services Agency for Healthcare
Research and Quality
www.ahrq.gov

Canadian Healthcare Education Commons / Collaboration pour
l'éducation en santé au Canada (CHEC-CESC)
http://chec-cesc.afmc.ca

Recommended Reading

Alexander M, Lenahan P, Pavlov A, eds. *Cinemeducation: A Comprehensive Guide to Using Film in Medical Education*. London: Radcliffe Publishing Ltd; 2005.

Alexander M, Lenahan P, Pavlov A, eds. *Cinemeducation: Using Film and Other Visual Media in Graduate and Medical Education*, vol. 2. London: Radcliffe Publishing Ltd; 2005.

Alguire PC. *Teaching in Your Office: A Guide to Instructing Medical Students & Residents*. 2nd ed. Philadelphia: American College of Physicians; 2010.

Anderson J, Barnes E, Shackleton E. *The Art of Medicine: Over 2,000 Years of Images and Imagination*. Chicago: University of Chicago Press; 2012.

Bleakley A. *Medical Humanities and Medical Education: How the Medical Humanities Can Shape Better Doctors*. New York: Routledge; 2015.

Bonebakker V, Naelhaft RL, eds. *Imagine What It's Like: A Literature and Medicine Anthology*. Honolulu: University of Hawaii Press; 2008.

Bordin G. *Medicine in Art*. Los Angeles: Getty Publications; 2010.

Charon R. *Narrative Medicine: Honoring the Stories of Illness*. New York: Oxford University Press; 2008.

Crawford A, Peterkin A, et al., eds. *Body & Soul: Narratives of Healing from Ars Medica*. Toronto: University of Toronto Press; 2011.

Crawford P, et al. *Health Humanities*. London: Palgrave Macmillan; 2015.

Davis M, McKimm J, Forrest K. *How to Assess Doctors and Health Professionals*. London: BMJ Books; 2013. http://dx.doi.org/10.1002/9781118523469.

Dobson M. *The Story of Medicine: From Leeches to Gene Therapy*. London: Quercus; 2013.

Duffin J. *History of Medicine: A Scandalously Short Introduction*. 2nd ed. Toronto: University of Toronto Press; 2010.

Ende J. *Theory and Practice of Teaching Medicine*. Philadelphia: American College of Physicians; 2010.

Frank AW. *The Wounded Storyteller: Body, Illness, and Ethics*. 2nd ed. Chicago: University of Chicago Press; 2013.

Gawande A. *Being Mortal*. Toronto: Doubleday Canada; 2014.

Halpern J. *From Detached Concern to Empathy – Humanizing Medical Practice*. Oxford: Oxford University Press; 2001. http://dx.doi.org/10.1093/acprof:osobl/9780195111194.001.0001.

Hammond MM, Kim S, eds. *Rethinking Empathy through Literature*. New York: Routledge; 2014.

Harden RM, Laidlaw JM. *Essential Skills for a Medical Teacher: An Introduction to Teaching and Learning in Medicine*. London: Churchill Livingstone; 2012.

Harvey BJ, Lang ES, Frank JR. *The Research Guide: A Primer for Residents, Other Health Care Trainees, and Practitioners*. Ottawa: Royal College of Physicians and Surgeons of Canada; 2011.

Humphrey H. *Mentoring in Academic Medicine*. Philadelphia: American College of Physicians; 2010.

Inhorn MC, Wentzell EA, editors. *Medical Anthropology at the Intersections: Histories, Activisms, and Futures*. Durham: Duke University Press; 2012. http://dx.doi.org/10.1215/9780822395478.

Jamison L. *The Empathy Exams: Essays*. Minneapolis: Graywolf Press; 2014.

Jones T, Wear D, Friedman LD, eds. *Health Humanities Reader*. New Brunswick, NJ: Rutgers University Press, 2014.

Klass P. *Treatment Kind and Fair: Letters to a Young Doctor*. New York: Basic Books; 2008.

Kleinman A. *The Illness Narratives: Suffering, Healing, and the Human Condition*. New York: Basic Books; 1989.

Nussbaum M. *Not for Profit – Why Democracy Needs the Humanities*. Princeton: Princeton University Press; 2010.

Oatley K. *Such Stuff as Dreams: The Psychology of Fiction*. New York: Wiley; 2011. http://dx.doi.org/10.1002/9781119970910.

Pangaro L. *Leadership Careers in Medical Education*. Philadelphia: American College of Physicians; 2010.

Schleifer R, Vannatta J, Chow S. *The Chief Concern of Medicine: The Integration of the Medical Humanities and Narrative Knowledge into Medical Practices*. Ann Arbor: University of Michigan Press; 2013.

Selzer R. *Letters to a Young Doctor*. New York: Mariner Books; 2013.

Singer M, Erickson PI, eds. *A Companion to Medical Anthropology*. Chichester, West Sussex: Wiley-Blackwell; 2015.

Skeff K. *Methods for Teaching Medicine*. Philadelphia: American College of Physicians; 2010.

Small H. *The Value of the Humanities*. Oxford: Oxford University Press; 2013. http://dx.doi.org/10.1093/acprof:oso/9780199683864.001.0001.

CHAPTER NINE

Bioethics Websites

American Medical Association Virtual Mentor
http://virtualmentor.ama-assn.org

American Society of Bioethics and Humanities
www.asbh.org

Canadian Bioethics Society
www.bioethics.ca
(Both the ASBH and CBS websites contain useful links and up-to-date bibliographies.)

The Hastings Center Report (journal)
See also www.thehastingscenter.org

Kennedy Institute of Ethics
https://bioethics.georgetown.edu

The Physician Litigation Stress Resource Center
www.physicianlitigationstress.org

Royal College of Physicians and Surgeons of Canada – Bioethics Project
http://www.royalcollege.ca/portal/page/portal/rc/resources/bioethics

University of British Columbia Library, Bioethicsline
http://resources.library.ubc.ca/263

University of Washington School of Medicine, Bioethics Resources
https://depts.washington.edu/bioethx/topics

Legal Resources

Canada

Canadian Medical Protective Association
https://www.cmpa-acpm.ca/home

United States

American Medical Association
http://www.ama-assn.org/ama

Physician Litigation Stress Resource Center
http://physicianlitigationstress.org

Contact your local union, housestaff association, AMA chapter, or hospital legal department.

Recommended Reading

Brenner IR. *How to Survive a Medical Malpractice Lawsuit: The Physician's Roadmap for Success*. London: BMJ Books; 2011.

Hafferty FW, Franks R. The hidden curriculum, ethics teaching and the structure of medical education. *Acad Med*. 1994; 69:861–71.

Levinson W, Ginsburg S, Hafferty FW, et al. *Understanding Medical Professionalism*. New York: McGraw-Hill Professional; 2014.

McCarthy M. *The Real Doctor Will See You Shortly: A Physician's First Year*. New York: Crown Publishing Group; 2015.

Mitchell DE, Ream RK, eds. *Professional Responsibility: The Fundamental Issue in Education and Health Care Reform*. Cham: Springer; 2015. http://dx.doi.org/10.1007/978-3-319-02603-9.

O'Reilly JT, Young ML. *Medical Malpractice: Avoiding, Adjudicating & Litigating in the Challenging New Climate*. Chicago: American Bar Association; 2015.

Pellegrino ED, Engelhart HT Jr, Jotterand F, eds. *The Philosophy of Medicine Reborn: A Pellegrino Reader*. Notre Dame: University of Notre Dame Press; 2008.

Pellegrino ED, Schulman A, Merrill TW. *Human Dignity and Bioethics*. Notre Dame: University of Notre Dame Press; 2009.

Pellegrino ED, Thomasma DC. *The Virtues in Medical Practice*. New York: Oxford University Press; 1993.

Singer PA, Viens AM (eds). *The Cambridge Textbook of Bioethics*. Cambridge: Cambridge University Press; 2008.

Wachter R. *The Digital Doctor: Hope, Hype, and Harm at the Dawn of Medicine's Computer Age*. New York: McGraw-Hill; 2015.

CHAPTER TEN

Financial and Business Resources

Canada

MD Management Limited
https://mdm.ca

MD Management and the CMA publish a guide called New in Practice – What Medical Residents Need to Know before Entering Practice (Ottawa, issued yearly).

United States

AMA–Resident Physician Section re: Practice Management Workshops
http://www.ama-assn.org/ama

AMA publishes a very helpful document called "Succeeding from Medical School to Practice."
http://www.ama-assn.org/ama/pub/about-ama/our-people/
member-groups-sections/resident-fellow-section/succeeding-
medical-school-practice.page

Check also with your specialty association for information on seminars and resources.

Recommended Reading

American Medical Association. *Starting Owning and Buying a Medical Practice*. Washington: American Medical Association; 2015.

Canadian Medical Association. *New in Practice*. Ottawa: CMA; 2015.

CHAPTER ELEVEN

The Resilient Physician (www.The Resilient Physician.com; 1-888-629-2313), a bimonthly newsletter "dedicated to today's physicians, medical families, and medical organizations," contains practical tips on improving the quality of life for doctors and their patients.

Recommended Conferences

The CMA (Canadian Medical Association), AMA (American Medical Association), and BMA (British Medical Association) hold an International Conference on Physician Health every 2 years. Visit their websites for further information.

National Medical Associations

American Medical Association
http://www.ama-assn.org/ama

Canadian Medical Association
https://www.cma.ca

International Medical Associations

British Medical Association
http://bma.org.uk

Commonwealth Medical Trust
http://ngosbeyond2014.org

Pan American Health Organization
www.paho.org

Pan American Medical Association
http://pamacfl.org

World Health Organization
www.who.int/en

World Medical Association
http://www.wma.net/en/10home/index.html

Special Interest Groups

Please refer to the July and January online issues of the current year of the *Journal of the American Medical Association* for the most recent web addresses of these and hundreds of other groups of interest and for new annual conference dates:

American Medical Women's Association
Christian Medical and Dental Society
Doctors Without Borders
Gay and Lesbian Medical Association
National Library of Medicine

Recommended Reading

Askin E, Moore N. *Health Care Handbook: A Clear and Concise Guide to the United States Healthcare System*. St Louis: Washington University; 2014.

Clarke F, Slavin L. *How to Manage Your GP Practice*. London: BMJ Books; 2011. http://dx.doi.org/10.1002/9781119959564.

Cooke M, Irby DM, O'Brien BC. *Education Physicians: A Call for Reform of Medical School and Residency*. San Francisco: Jossey-Bass; 2010.

Davis M, McKimm J, Forrest K. *How to Assess Doctors and Health Professionals*. London: BMJ Books; 2013. http://dx.doi.org/10.1002/9781118523469.

Dent J, Harden RM, eds. *A Practical Guide for Medical Teachers*. 4th ed. London: Churchill Livingstone; 2013.

Donhoe M, ed. *Public Health and Social Justice*. San Francisco: Jossey-Bass; 2012.

John E. *Building on the Best: An Introduction to Appreciative Inquiry in Healthcare*. Chichester: Kingsham Press; 2006.

Eisenberg MJ. *The Physician Scientist's Career Guide*. New York: Springer; 2011. http://dx.doi.org/10.1007/978-1-60327-908-6.

Ende J. *Theory and Practice of Teaching Medicine*. Philadelphia: American College of Physicians; 2010.

Farmer P, Kleinman A, Kim JY, et al., editors. *Reimagining Global Health: An Introduction*. Oakland: University of California Press; 2013.

Forman D, Jones M, Thistlethwaite J, eds. *Leadership Development for Interprofessional Education and Collaborative Practice*. London: Palgrave Macmillan; 2014. http://dx.doi.org/10.1057/9781137363022.

Goldman LS, ed. *The Handbook of Physician Health: The Essential Guide to Understanding the Health Care Needs of Physicians*. Chicago: AMA Press; 2000.

Goodman NW, Edwards MB, Black A. *Medical Writing: A Prescription for Clarity*. 4th ed. Cambridge: Cambridge University Press; 2014. http://dx.doi.org/10.1017/CBO9781107279179.

Guest C, Ricciardi W, Kawachi I, et al., eds. *Oxford Handbook of Public Health Practice*. 3rd ed. Oxford University Press; 2013. http://dx.doi.org/10.1093/med/9780199586301.001.0001.

Guerrasio J. *Remediation of the Struggling Medical Learner*. Irwin, PA: Association for Hospital Medical Education; 2013.

Hafferty FW, O'Donnell JF, eds. *The Hidden Curriculum in Health Professional Education*. Hanover: Dartmouth College Press, 2015.

Harden RM, Laidlaw JM. *Essential Skills for a Medical Teacher: An Introduction to Teaching and Learning in Medicine*. London: Churchill Livingstone; 2012.

Huggett K, Jeffries WB, eds. *An Introduction to Medical Teaching*. 2nd ed. Dordrecht: Springer; 2014. http://dx.doi.org/10.1007/978-94-017-9066-6.

Humphrey H. *Mentoring in Academic Medicine*. Philadelphia: American College of Physicians; 2010.

Kaminsky L, ed. *Writer M.D: The Best Contemporary Fiction and Nonfiction by Doctors*. New York: Vintage; 2012.

Lueddeke GR. *Transforming Medical Education for the 21st Century: Megatrends, Priorities and Change*. London: Radcliffe Medical Press; 2012.

MacCarrick G. *Medical Leadership and Management: A Case-based Approach*. London: Springer; 2014.

Moawad HG. *Careers beyond Clinical Medicine*. New York: Oxford
University Press; 2012.

Nelson S, Tassone M, Hodges B. *Creating the Health Care Team of the
Future: The Toronto Model for Interprofessional Education and Practice*.
Ithaca, NY: ILR Press; 2014.

New in Practice. Ottawa: Canadian Medical Association; 2014.

Pangaro L. *Leadership Careers in Medical Education*. Philadelphia:
American College of Physicians; 2010.

Roberts LW, ed. *The Academic Medicine Handbook: A Guide to
Achievement and Fulfillment for Academic Faculty*. New York:
Springer; 2013. http://dx.doi.org/10.1007/978-1-4614-5693-3.

Schroeder K, Thompson T, Frith K, et al. *Sustainable Healthcare*.
London: BMJ Books; 2013.

Skeff K. *Methods for Teaching Medicine*. Philadelphia: American College
of Physicians; 2010.

Steinert Y, ed. *Faculty Development in the Health Professions: A Focus
on Research and Practice*. Dordrecht: Springer; 2014. http://dx.doi.
org/10.1007/978-94-007-7612-8.

Straus S, Sackett D. *Mentorship in Academic Medicine*. London: BMJ
Books; 2013. http://dx.doi.org/10.1002/9781118446065.

Swanwick T, ed. *Understanding Medical Education: Evidence, Theory and
Practice*. 2nd ed. West Sussex: Wiley-Blackwell; 2013. http://dx.doi.
org/10.1002/9781118472361.

CHAPTER TWELVE

Recommended Reading – How to Assess Online Articles

Greenhalgh T. *How to Read a Paper: The Basics of Evidence-Based
Medicine*. 5th ed. London: BMJ Books; 2014.

Guyatt G. *User's Guides to the Medical Literature: A Manual for Evidence-
based Clinical Practice*. 3rd ed. New York: McGraw-Hill Professional;
2014.

Index

From the author of *Staying Human during Residency Training*

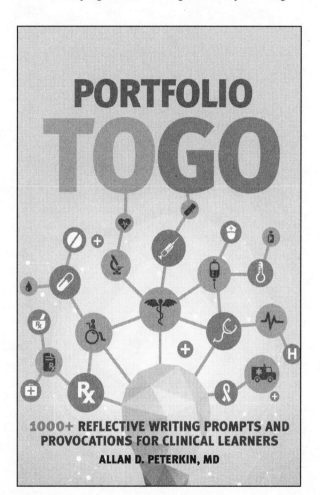

How can health professionals develop their reflective capacity, critical thinking, creative expression, and narrative competence? In his new book *Portfolio to Go*, Allan D. Peterkin presents over 1000 novel and clinically relevant reflective writing prompts for undergraduate and post-graduate clinical learners across a wide variety of healthcare professions.

utppublishing.com